THE OFFICIAL PATIENT'S SOURCEBOOK

on

SHOULDER SEPARATION

JAMES N. PARKER, M.D.
AND PHILIP M. PARKER, PH.D., EDITORS

ICON Health Publications
ICON Group International, Inc.
4370 La Jolla Village Drive, 4th Floor
San Diego, CA 92122 USA

Printed in the United States of America.

Last digit indicates print number: 10 9 8 7 6 4 5 3 2 1

Publisher, Health Care: Tiffany LaRochelle
Editor(s): James Parker, M.D., Philip Parker, Ph.D.

Publisher's note: The ideas, procedures, and suggestions contained in this book are not intended as a substitute for consultation with your physician. All matters regarding your health require medical supervision. As new medical or scientific information becomes available from academic and clinical research, recommended treatments and drug therapies may undergo changes. The authors, editors, and publisher have attempted to make the information in this book up to date and accurate in accord with accepted standards at the time of publication. The authors, editors, and publisher are not responsible for errors or omissions or for consequences from application of the book, and make no warranty, expressed or implied, in regard to the contents of this book. Any practice described in this book should be applied by the reader in accordance with professional standards of care used in regard to the unique circumstances that may apply in each situation, in close consultation with a qualified physician. The reader is advised to always check product information (package inserts) for changes and new information regarding dose and contraindications before taking any drug or pharmacological product. Caution is especially urged when using new or infrequently ordered drugs, herbal remedies, vitamins and supplements, alternative therapies, complementary therapies and medicines, and integrative medical treatments.

Cataloging-in-Publication Data

Parker, James N., 1961-
Parker, Philip M., 1960-

The Official Patient's Sourcebook on Shoulder Separation: A Revised and Updated Directory for the Internet Age/James N. Parker and Philip M. Parker, editors
     p.   cm.
Includes bibliographical references, glossary and index.
ISBN: 0-597-83176-9
1. Shoulder Separation-Popular works.   I. Title.

Disclaimer

This publication is not intended to be used for the diagnosis or treatment of a health problem or as a substitute for consultation with licensed medical professionals. It is sold with the understanding that the publisher, editors, and authors are not engaging in the rendering of medical, psychological, financial, legal, or other professional services.

References to any entity, product, service, or source of information that may be contained in this publication should not be considered an endorsement, either direct or implied, by the publisher, editors or authors. ICON Group International, Inc., the editors, or the authors are not responsible for the content of any Web pages nor publications referenced in this publication.

Copyright Notice

Dedication

To the healthcare professionals dedicating their time and efforts to the study of shoulder separation.

Acknowledgements

The collective knowledge generated from academic and applied research summarized in various references has been critical in the creation of this sourcebook which is best viewed as a comprehensive compilation and collection of information prepared by various official agencies which directly or indirectly are dedicated to the study of shoulder separation. All of the *Official Patient's Sourcebooks* draw from various agencies and institutions associated with the United States Department of Health and Human Services, and in particular, the Office of the Secretary of Health and Human Services (OS), the Administration for Children and Families (ACF), the Administration on Aging (AOA), the Agency for Healthcare Research and Quality (AHRQ), the Agency for Toxic Substances and Disease Registry (ATSDR), the Centers for Disease Control and Prevention (CDC), the Food and Drug Administration (FDA), the Healthcare Financing Administration (HCFA), the Health Resources and Services Administration (HRSA), the Indian Health Service (IHS), the institutions of the National Institutes of Health (NIH), the Program Support Center (PSC), and the Substance Abuse and Mental Health Services Administration (SAMHSA). In addition to these sources, information gathered from the National Library of Medicine, the United States Patent Office, the European Union, and their related organizations has been invaluable in the creation of this sourcebook. Some of the work represented was financially supported by the Research and Development Committee at INSEAD. This support is gratefully acknowledged. Finally, special thanks are owed to Tiffany LaRochelle for her excellent editorial support.

About the Editors

James N. Parker, M.D.

Dr. James N. Parker received his Bachelor of Science degree in Psychobiology from the University of California, Riverside and his M.D. from the University of California, San Diego. In addition to authoring numerous research publications, he has lectured at various academic institutions. Dr. Parker is the medical editor for the *Official Patient's Sourcebook* series published by ICON Health Publications.

Philip M. Parker, Ph.D.

Philip M. Parker is the Eli Lilly Chair Professor of Innovation, Business and Society at INSEAD (Fontainebleau, France and Singapore). Dr. Parker has also been Professor at the University of California, San Diego and has taught courses at Harvard University, the Hong Kong University of Science and Technology, the Massachusetts Institute of Technology, Stanford University, and UCLA. Dr. Parker is the associate editor for the *Official Patient's Sourcebook* series published by ICON Health Publications.

About ICON Health Publications

In addition to shoulder separation, *Official Patient's Sourcebooks* are available for the following related topics:

- The Official Patient's Sourcebook on Arthritis of the Shoulder
- The Official Patient's Sourcebook on Frozen Shoulder
- The Official Patient's Sourcebook on Rotator Cuff Injury
- The Official Patient's Sourcebook on Shoulder Bursitis
- The Official Patient's Sourcebook on Shoulder Dislocation
- The Official Patient's Sourcebook on Shoulder Fracture
- The Official Patient's Sourcebook on Shoulder Impingement Syndrome
- The Official Patient's Sourcebook on Shoulder Tendinitis
- The Official Patient's Sourcebook on Wrist Sprains and Strains

To discover more about ICON Health Publications, simply check with your preferred online booksellers, including Barnes & Noble.com and Amazon.com which currently carry all of our titles. Or, feel free to contact us directly for bulk purchases or institutional discounts:

ICON Group International, Inc.
4370 La Jolla Village Drive, Fourth Floor
San Diego, CA 92122 USA
Fax: 858-546-4341
Web site: **www.icongrouponline.com/health**

Table of Contents

INTRODUCTION..1
   Overview..1
   Organization...3
   Scope..3
   Moving Forward...4

PART I: THE ESSENTIALS..7

CHAPTER 1. THE ESSENTIALS ON SHOULDER SEPARATION: GUIDELINES..9
   Overview..9
   How Common Are Shoulder Problems?..10
   What Are the Structures of the Shoulder and How Does It Function?.........11
   What Are the Origin and Causes of Shoulder Problems?............................12
   How Are Shoulder Problems Diagnosed?...12
   What Is Shoulder Separation?...13
   What Are the Signs of Shoulder Separation and How Is It Diagnosed?....13
   How Is Shoulder Separation Treated?...13
   Where Can I Get Additional Information about Shoulder Problems?........14
   More Guideline Sources..15
   Vocabulary Builder..18

CHAPTER 2. SEEKING GUIDANCE..21
   Overview...21
   Associations and Shoulder Separation..21
   Finding Doctors...23
   Finding an Orthopedic Surgeon..25
   Selecting Your Doctor...25
   Working with Your Doctor...26
   Broader Health-Related Resources...27

PART II: ADDITIONAL RESOURCES AND ADVANCED MATERIAL..29

CHAPTER 3. STUDIES ON SHOULDER SEPARATION....................31
   Overview...31
   The Combined Health Information Database...31
   The National Library of Medicine: PubMed..32
   Vocabulary Builder..33

CHAPTER 4. BOOKS ON SHOULDER SEPARATION......................35
   Overview...35
   Book Summaries: Online Booksellers...35
   The National Library of Medicine Book Index..35

Chapters on Shoulder Separation..40
General Home References..40
Vocabulary Builder..41

CHAPTER 5. MULTIMEDIA ON SHOULDER SEPARATION..........43
Overview..43
Bibliography: Multimedia on Shoulder Separation..43
Vocabulary Builder..47

PART III. APPENDICES..49

APPENDIX A. RESEARCHING YOUR MEDICATIONS..........51
Overview..51
Your Medications: The Basics..52
Learning More about Your Medications..54
Commercial Databases..54
Contraindications and Interactions (Hidden Dangers)..........................55
A Final Warning..56
General References..57

APPENDIX B. RESEARCHING NUTRITION..........59
Overview..59
Food and Nutrition: General Principles..60
Finding Studies on Shoulder Separation..64
Federal Resources on Nutrition..65
Additional Web Resources..66
Vocabulary Builder..67

APPENDIX C. FINDING MEDICAL LIBRARIES..........69
Overview..69
Preparation..69
Finding a Local Medical Library..70
Medical Libraries Open to the Public..70

APPENDIX D. CHILDHOOD SPORTS INJURIES AND THEIR PREVENTION..........77
Overview..77
Childhood Sports Injuries and Their Prevention..........................77
Treat Injuries with "RICE"..78
Heat and Hydration - Playing It Safe Is Cool..79
Sports Injury and Prevention..80
How Your Child Can Prevent Sports Injuries..82
Additional Resources..83
Vocabulary Builder..84

ONLINE GLOSSARIES..87
Online Dictionary Directories..88

SHOULDER SEPARATION GLOSSARY............................89

    General Dictionaries and Glossaries 94

INDEX...96

INTRODUCTION

Overview

Dr. C. Everett Koop, former U.S. Surgeon General, once said, "The best prescription is knowledge."[1] The Agency for Healthcare Research and Quality (AHRQ) of the National Institutes of Health (NIH) echoes this view and recommends that every patient incorporate education into the treatment process. According to the AHRQ:

> Finding out more about your condition is a good place to start. By contacting groups that support your condition, visiting your local library, and searching on the Internet, you can find good information to help guide your treatment decisions. Some information may be hard to find — especially if you don't know where to look.[2]

As the AHRQ mentions, finding the right information is not an obvious task. Though many physicians and public officials had thought that the emergence of the Internet would do much to assist patients in obtaining reliable information, in March 2001 the National Institutes of Health issued the following warning:

> The number of Web sites offering health-related resources grows every day. Many sites provide valuable information, while others may have information that is unreliable or misleading.[3]

---

[1] Quotation from http://www.drkoop.com.
[2] The Agency for Healthcare Research and Quality (AHRQ):
http://www.ahcpr.gov/consumer/diaginfo.htm.
[3] From the NIH, National Cancer Institute (NCI):
http://cancertrials.nci.nih.gov/beyond/evaluating.html.

Since the late 1990s, physicians have seen a general increase in patient Internet usage rates. Patients frequently enter their doctor's offices with printed Web pages of home remedies in the guise of latest medical research. This scenario is so common that doctors often spend more time dispelling misleading information than guiding patients through sound therapies. *The Official Patient's Sourcebook on Shoulder Separation* has been created for patients who have decided to make education and research an integral part of the treatment process. The pages that follow will tell you where and how to look for information covering virtually all topics related to shoulder separation, from the essentials to the most advanced areas of research.

The title of this book includes the word "official." This reflects the fact that the sourcebook draws from public, academic, government, and peer-reviewed research. Selected readings from various agencies are reproduced to give you some of the latest official information available to date on shoulder separation.

Given patients' increasing sophistication in using the Internet, abundant references to reliable Internet-based resources are provided throughout this sourcebook. Where possible, guidance is provided on how to obtain free-of-charge, primary research results as well as more detailed information via the Internet. E-book and electronic versions of this sourcebook are fully interactive with each of the Internet sites mentioned (clicking on a hyperlink automatically opens your browser to the site indicated). Hard copy users of this sourcebook can type cited Web addresses directly into their browsers to obtain access to the corresponding sites. Since we are working with ICON Health Publications, hard copy *Sourcebooks* are frequently updated and printed on demand to ensure that the information provided is current.

In addition to extensive references accessible via the Internet, every chapter presents a "Vocabulary Builder." Many health guides offer glossaries of technical or uncommon terms in an appendix. In editing this sourcebook, we have decided to place a smaller glossary within each chapter that covers terms used in that chapter. Given the technical nature of some chapters, you may need to revisit many sections. Building one's vocabulary of medical terms in such a gradual manner has been shown to improve the learning process.

We must emphasize that no sourcebook on shoulder separation should affirm that a specific diagnostic procedure or treatment discussed in a research study, patent, or doctoral dissertation is "correct" or your best option. This sourcebook is no exception. Each patient is unique. Deciding on appropriate options is always up to the patient in consultation with their physician and healthcare providers.

Organization

This sourcebook is organized into three parts. Part I explores basic techniques to researching shoulder separation (e.g. finding guidelines on diagnosis, treatments, and prognosis), followed by a number of topics, including information on how to get in touch with organizations, associations, or other patient networks dedicated to shoulder separation. It also gives you sources of information that can help you find a doctor in your local area specializing in diagnosing and treating shoulder separation. Collectively, the material presented in Part I is a complete primer on basic research topics for patients with shoulder separation.

Part II moves on to advanced research dedicated to shoulder separation. Part II is intended for those willing to invest many hours of hard work and study. It is here that we direct you to the latest scientific and applied research on shoulder separation. When possible, contact names, links via the Internet, and summaries are provided. It is in Part II where the vocabulary process becomes important as authors publishing advanced research frequently use highly specialized language. In general, every attempt is made to recommend "free-to-use" options.

Part III provides appendices of useful background reading for all patients with shoulder separation or related injuries. The appendices are dedicated to more pragmatic issues faced by many patients with shoulder separation. Accessing materials via medical libraries may be the only option for some readers, so a guide is provided for finding local medical libraries which are open to the public. Part III, therefore, focuses on advice that goes beyond the biological and scientific issues facing patients with shoulder separation.

Scope

While this sourcebook covers shoulder separation, your doctor, research publications, and specialists may refer to your condition using a variety of terms. Therefore, you should understand that shoulder separation is often considered a synonym or a condition closely related to the following:

- Fracture of the Shoulder
- Shoulder Separation

In addition to synonyms and related conditions, physicians may refer to shoulder separation using certain coding systems. The International Classification of Diseases, 9th Revision, Clinical Modification (ICD-9-CM) is the most commonly used system of classification for the world's illnesses. Your physician may use this coding system as an administrative or tracking tool. The following classification is commonly used for shoulder separation:[4]

For the purposes of this sourcebook, we have attempted to be as inclusive as possible, looking for official information for all of the synonyms relevant to shoulder separation. You may find it useful to refer to synonyms when accessing databases or interacting with healthcare professionals and medical librarians.

Moving Forward

Since the 1980s, the world has seen a proliferation of healthcare guides covering most illnesses and conditions. Some are written by patients or their family members. These generally take a layperson's approach to understanding and coping with an illness or injury. They can be uplifting, encouraging, and highly supportive. Other guides are authored by physicians or other healthcare providers who have a more clinical outlook. Each of these two styles of guide has its purpose and can be quite useful.

As editors, we have chosen a third route. We have chosen to expose you to as many sources of official and peer-reviewed information as practical, for the purpose of educating you about basic and advanced knowledge as recognized by medical science today. You can think of this sourcebook as your personal Internet age reference librarian.

Why "Internet age"? All too often, patients with shoulder separation will log on to the Internet, type words into a search engine, and receive several Web site listings which are mostly irrelevant or redundant. These patients are left to wonder where the relevant information is, and how to obtain it. Since only the smallest fraction of information dealing with shoulder separation is even indexed in search engines, a non-systematic approach often leads to frustration and disappointment. With this sourcebook, we hope to direct you

---

[4] This list is based on the official version of the World Health Organization's 9th Revision, International Classification of Diseases (ICD-9). According to the National Technical Information Service, "ICD-9CM extensions, interpretations, modifications, addenda, or errata other than those approved by the U.S. Public Health Service and the Health Care Financing Administration are not to be considered official and should not be utilized. Continuous maintenance of the ICD-9-CM is the responsibility of the federal government."

to the information you need that you would not likely find using popular Web directories. Beyond Web listings, in many cases we will reproduce brief summaries or abstracts of available reference materials. These abstracts often contain distilled information on topics of discussion.

Before beginning your search for information, it is important for you to realize that shoulder separation is considered a relatively uncommon condition. Because of this, far less research is conducted on shoulder separation compared to other health problems afflicting larger populations, like breast cancer or heart disease. Nevertheless, this sourcebook will prove useful for two reasons. First, if more information does become available on shoulder separation, the sources given in this book will be the most likely to report or make such information available. Second, some will find it important to know about patient support, symptom management, or diagnostic procedures that may be relevant to both shoulder separation and other conditions. By using the sources listed in the following chapters, self-directed research can be conducted on broader topics that are related to shoulder separation but not readily uncovered using general Internet search engines (e.g. www.google.com or www.yahoo.com). In this way, we have designed this sourcebook to complement these general search engines that can provide useful information and access to online patient support groups.[5]

While we focus on the more scientific aspects of shoulder separation, there is, of course, the emotional side to consider. Later in the sourcebook, we provide a chapter dedicated to helping you find peer groups and associations that can provide additional support beyond research produced by medical science. We hope that the choices we have made give you the most options available in moving forward. In this way, we wish you the best in your efforts to incorporate this educational approach into your treatment plan.

The Editors

---

[5] For example, one can simply go to **www.google.com,** or other general search engines (e.g. **www.yahoo.com** , **www.aol.com,** **www.msn.com**) and type in "diseasex support group" to find any active online support groups dedicated to diseasex.

PART I: THE ESSENTIALS

ABOUT PART I

Part I has been edited to give you access to what we feel are "the essentials" on shoulder separation. The essentials of an injury typically include the definition or description of the injury, a discussion of who it affects, the symptoms that are associated with a given injury, tests or diagnostic procedures that might be specific to the injury, and treatments for the injury. Your doctor or healthcare provider may have already explained the essentials of shoulder separation to you or even given you a pamphlet or brochure describing shoulder separation. Now you are searching for more in-depth information. As editors, we have decided, nevertheless, to include a discussion on where to find essential information that can complement what your doctor has already told you. In this section we recommend a process, not a particular Web site or reference book. The process ensures that, as you search the Web, you gain background information in such a way as to maximize your understanding.

CHAPTER 1. THE ESSENTIALS ON SHOULDER SEPARATION: GUIDELINES

Overview

Official agencies, as well as federally-funded institutions supported by national grants, frequently publish a variety of guidelines on shoulder separation. These are typically called "Fact Sheets" or "Guidelines." They can take the form of a brochure, information kit, pamphlet, or flyer. Often they are only a few pages in length. The great advantage of guidelines over other sources is that they are often written with the patient in mind. Since new guidelines on shoulder separation can appear at any moment and be published by a number of sources, the best approach to finding guidelines is to systematically scan the Internet-based services that post them.

The National Institutes of Health (NIH)[6]

The National Institutes of Health (NIH) is the first place to search for relatively current patient guidelines and fact sheets on shoulder separation. Originally founded in 1887, the NIH is one of the world's foremost medical research centers and the federal focal point for medical research in the United States. At any given time, the NIH supports some 35,000 research grants at universities, medical schools, and other research and training institutions, both nationally and internationally. The rosters of those who have conducted research or who have received NIH support over the years include the world's most illustrious scientists and physicians. Among them are 97 scientists who have won the Nobel Prize for achievement in medicine.

---

[6] Adapted from the NIH: **http://www.nih.gov/about/NIHoverview.html**.

There is no guarantee that any one Institute will have a guideline on a specific condition or disease, though the National Institutes of Health collectively publish over 600 guidelines for both common and rare conditions and disorders. The best way to access NIH guidelines is via the Internet. Although the NIH is organized into many different Institutes and Offices, the following is a list of key Web sites where you are most likely to find NIH clinical guidelines and publications dealing with shoulder separation and associated conditions:

- Office of the Director (OD); guidelines consolidated across agencies available at **http://www.nih.gov/health/consumer/conkey.htm**

- National Library of Medicine (NLM); extensive encyclopedia (A.D.A.M., Inc.) with guidelines available at **http://www.nlm.nih.gov/medlineplus/healthtopics.html**

- National Institute of Arthritis and Musculoskeletal and Skin Diseases (NIAMS); fact sheets and guidelines at **http://www.nih.gov/niams/healthinfo/**

Among those listed above, the National Institute of Arthritis and Musculoskeletal and Skin Diseases (NIAMS) is especially noteworthy. The mission of NIAMS, a part of the National Institutes of Health (NIH), is to support research into the causes, treatment, and prevention of arthritis and musculoskeletal and skin diseases, the training of basic and clinical scientists to carry out this research, and the dissemination of information on research progress in these diseases. The National Institute of Arthritis and Musculoskeletal and Skin Diseases Information Clearinghouse is a public service sponsored by the NIAMS that provides health information and information sources. The NIAMS provides the following guideline concerning shoulder separation .[7]

How Common Are Shoulder Problems?[8]

According to the American Academy of Orthopaedic Surgeons, about 4 million people in the United States seek medical care each year for shoulder sprain, strain, dislocation, or other problems. Each year, shoulder problems account for about 1.5 million visits to orthopaedic surgeons--doctors who treat disorders of the bones, muscles, and related structures.

---

[7] This and other passages are adapted from the NIH and NIAMS (**http://www.niams.nih.gov/hi/index.htm**). "Adapted" signifies that the text is reproduced with attribution, with some or no editorial adjustments.

[8] Adapted from the National Institute of Arthritis and Musculoskeletal and Skin Diseases (NIAMS): **http://www.niams.nih.gov/hi/topics/shoulderprobs/shoulderqa.htm** .

What Are the Structures of the Shoulder and How Does It Function?

The shoulder joint is composed of three bones: the clavicle (collarbone), the scapula (shoulder blade), and the humerus (upper arm bone) (see diagram). Two joints facilitate shoulder movement. The acromioclavicular (AC) joint is located between the acromion (part of the scapula that forms the highest point of the shoulder) and the clavicle. The glenohumeral joint, commonly called the shoulder joint, is a ball-and-socket type joint that helps move the shoulder forward and backward and allows the arm to rotate in a circular fashion or hinge out and up away from the body. (The "ball" is the top, rounded portion of the upper arm bone or humerus; the "socket," or glenoid, is a dish-shaped part of the outer edge of the scapula into which the ball fits.) The capsule is a soft tissue envelope that encircles the glenohumeral joint. It is lined by a thin, smooth synovial membrane.

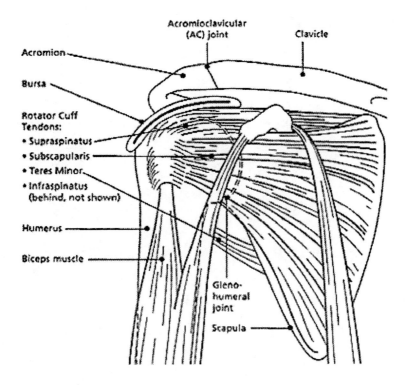

The bones of the shoulder are held in place by muscles, tendons, and ligaments. Tendons are tough cords of tissue that attach the shoulder muscles to bone and assist the muscles in moving the shoulder. Ligaments attach shoulder bones to each other, providing stability. For example, the front of the joint capsule is anchored by three glenohumeral ligaments.

The rotator cuff is a structure composed of tendons that, with associated muscles, holds the ball at the top of the humerus in the glenoid socket and provides mobility and strength to the shoulder joint.

Two filmy sac-like structures called bursae permit smooth gliding between bone, muscle, and tendon. They cushion and protect the rotator cuff from the bony arch of the acromion.

What Are the Origin and Causes of Shoulder Problems?

The shoulder is the most movable joint in the body. However, it is an unstable joint because of the range of motion allowed. It is easily subject to injury because the ball of the upper arm is larger than the shoulder socket that holds it. To remain stable, the shoulder must be anchored by its muscles, tendons, and ligaments. Some shoulder problems arise from the disruption of these soft tissues as a result of injury or from overuse or underuse of the shoulder. Other problems arise from a degenerative process in which tissues break down and no longer function well.

Shoulder pain may be localized or may be referred to areas around the shoulder or down the arm. Disease within the body (such as gallbladder, liver, or heart disease, or disease of the cervical spine of the neck) also may generate pain that travels along nerves to the shoulder.

How Are Shoulder Problems Diagnosed?

Following are some of the ways doctors diagnose shoulder problems:

- Medical history (the patient tells the doctor about an injury or other condition that might be causing the pain).
- Physical examination to feel for injury and discover the limits of movement, location of pain, and extent of joint instability.
- Diagnostic tests

Some of tests used to diagnose shoulder problems include:

- X ray
- Athrogram--Diagnostic record that can be seen on an x ray after injection of a contrast fluid into the shoulder joint to outline structures such as the rotator cuff. In disease or injury, this contrast fluid may either leak into

an area where it does not belong, indicating a tear or opening, or be blocked from entering an area where there normally is an opening.

- MRI (magnetic resonance imaging)--A non-invasive procedure in which a machine produces a series of cross-sectional images of the shoulder.

- Other diagnostic tests, such as injection of an anesthetic into and around the shoulder joint, are discussed in specific sections of this booklet.

What Is Shoulder Separation?

A shoulder separation occurs where the collarbone (clavicle) meets the shoulder blade (scapula). When ligaments that hold the joint together are partially or completely torn, the outer end of the clavicle may slip out of place, preventing it from properly meeting the scapula. Most often the injury is caused by a blow to the shoulder or by falling on an outstretched hand.

What Are the Signs of Shoulder Separation and How Is It Diagnosed?

Shoulder pain or tenderness and, occasionally, a bump in the middle of the top of the shoulder (over the AC joint) are signs that a separation may have occurred. Sometimes the severity of a separation can be detected by taking x rays while the patient holds a light weight that pulls on the muscles, making a separation more pronounced.

How Is Shoulder Separation Treated?

A shoulder separation is usually treated conservatively by rest and wearing a sling. Soon after injury, an ice bag may be applied to relieve pain and swelling. After a period of rest, a therapist helps the patient perform exercises that put the shoulder through its range of motion. Most shoulder separations heal within 2 or 3 months without further intervention. However, if ligaments are severely torn, surgical repair may be required to hold the clavicle in place. A doctor may wait to see if conservative treatment works before deciding whether surgery is required.

Where Can I Get Additional Information about Shoulder Problems?

For more information, contact:

National Institute of Arthritis and Musculoskeletal and Skin Diseases Information Clearinghouse
National Institutes of Health
1 AMS Circle
Bethesda, MD 20892-3675
Phone: 301-495-4484 or
877-22-NIAMS (226-4267) (free of charge)
TTY: 301-565-2966
Fax: 301-718-6366
http://www.niams.nih.gov/
The clearinghouse provides information about various forms of arthritis and rheumatic disease and bone, muscle, and skin diseases. It distributes patient and professional education materials and refers people to other sources of information. Additional information and updates can also be found on the NIAMS Web site.

American Academy of Orthopaedic Surgeons
P.O. Box 2058
Des Plaines, IL 60017
Phone: 800-824-BONE (2663) (free of charge)
Fax: 847-823-8025
www.aaos.org
The academy publishes brochures on total joint replacement, arthritis, arthroscopy, and other subjects. Single copies of a brochure are available free of charge by sending a self-addressed, stamped (business-size) envelope to *(name of brochure)* at the address above.

American College of Rheumatology
1800 Century Place, Suite 250
Atlanta, GA 30345
Phone: 404-633-3777
Fax: 404-633-1870
www.rheumatology.org
This national professional organization can provide referrals to rheumatologists and allied health specialists, such as physical therapists. One-page fact sheets are also available on various forms of arthritis. Lists of specialists by geographic area and fact sheets are also available on their Web site.

American Physical Therapy Association
1111 North Fairfax Street
Alexandria, VA 22314-1488
Phone: 703-684-2782 or
800-999-2782, ext. 3395 (free of charge)
www.apta.org
This national professional organization represents physical therapists, allied personnel, and students. Its objectives are to improve research, public understanding, and education in the physical therapies. A free brochure titled "Taking Care of Your Shoulder: A Physical Therapist's Perspective" is available on the association's Web site or by sending a business-size, stamped, self-addressed envelope to the address above.

Arthritis Foundation
1330 West Peachtree Street
Atlanta, GA 30309
Phone: 404-872-7100 or 800-283-7800 (free of charge)
or call your local chapter (listed in the telephone directory)
www.arthritis.org
This is the major voluntary organization devoted to arthritis. The foundation publishes pamphlets on arthritis, such as "Arthritis Answers," that may be obtained by calling the toll-free telephone number. The foundation also can provide physician and clinic referrals. Local chapters also provide information and organize exercise programs for people who have arthritis.

More Guideline Sources

The guideline above on shoulder separation is only one example of the kind of material that you can find online and free of charge. The remainder of this chapter will direct you to other sources which either publish or can help you find additional guidelines on topics related to shoulder separation. Many of the guidelines listed below address topics that may be of particular relevance to your specific situation or of special interest to only some patients with shoulder separation. Due to space limitations these sources are listed in a concise manner. Do not hesitate to consult the following sources by either using the Internet hyperlink provided, or, in cases where the contact information is provided, contacting the publisher or author directly.

Topic Pages: MEDLINEplus

For patients wishing to go beyond guidelines published by specific Institutes of the NIH, the National Library of Medicine has created a vast and patient-oriented healthcare information portal called MEDLINEplus. Within this Internet-based system are "health topic pages." You can think of a health topic page as a guide to patient guides. To access this system, log on to **http://www.nlm.nih.gov/medlineplus/healthtopics.html**.

If you do not find topics of interest when browsing health topic pages, then you can choose to use the advanced search utility of MEDLINEplus at **http://www.nlm.nih.gov/medlineplus/advancedsearch.html**. This utility is similar to the NIH Search Utility, with the exception that it only includes material linked within the MEDLINEplus system (mostly patient-oriented information). It also has the disadvantage of generating unstructured results. We recommend, therefore, that you use this method only if you have a very targeted search.

The National Guideline Clearinghouse™

The National Guideline Clearinghouse™ offers hundreds of evidence-based clinical practice guidelines published in the United States and other countries. You can search their site located at **http://www.guideline.gov** by using the keyword "shoulder separation" or synonyms. The following was recently posted:

- **AAOS clinical guideline on shoulder pain.**

    Source: American Academy of Orthopaedic Surgeons/American Academy of Physical Medicine and Rehabilitation/American College of Emergency Physicians/American College of Rheumatology.; 2001; 24 pages

    http://www.guideline.gov/FRAMESETS/guideline_fs.asp?guideline=002224&sSearch_string=shoulder+separation

Healthfinder™

Healthfinder™ is an additional source sponsored by the U.S. Department of Health and Human Services which offers links to hundreds of other sites that contain healthcare information. This Web site is located at

http://www.healthfinder.gov. Again, keyword searches can be used to find guidelines. The following was recently found in this database:

- **Common Peripartum Emergencies**

    Summary: A review of four types of common emergencies during labor and delivery: nonreassuring fetal status, maternal hemorrhage, fetal shoulder dystocia and eclampsia.

    Source: American Academy of Family Physicians

    http://www.healthfinder.gov/scripts/recordpass.asp?RecordType=0&RecordID=4247

- **FAQ - About Ankylosing Spondylitis (AS)**

    Summary: Online answers to consumers most commonly asked questions concerning this chronic, inflammatory condition that usually involves primarily the spine and joints of the extremities (such as shoulders,

    Source: Spondylitis Association of America

    http://www.healthfinder.gov/scripts/recordpass.asp?RecordType=0&RecordID=2155

- **Patient Guide to Shoulder Surgeries and Injuries**

    Summary: This patient education booklet describes types of shoulder surgeries and injuries including impingement, recurrent dislocation, painful instability and problems caused by musculoskeletal diseases.

    Source: Educational Institution--Follow the Resource URL for More Information

    http://www.healthfinder.gov/scripts/recordpass.asp?RecordType=0&RecordID=4094

- **Questions and Answers About Shoulder Problems**

    Summary: This fact sheet presents a general overview of the shoulder and shoulder problems as well as answers questions about specific shoulder problems (dislocation, separation, tendonitis, bursitis,

    Source: National Institute of Arthritis and Musculoskeletal and Skin Diseases, National Institutes of Health

    http://www.healthfinder.gov/scripts/recordpass.asp?RecordType=0&RecordID=5655

The NIH Search Utility

After browsing the references listed at the beginning of this chapter, you may want to explore the NIH Search Utility. This allows you to search for documents on over 100 selected Web sites that comprise the NIH-WEB-SPACE. Each of these servers is "crawled" and indexed on an ongoing basis. Your search will produce a list of various documents, all of which will relate in some way to shoulder separation. The drawbacks of this approach are that the information is not organized by theme and that the references are often a mix of information for professionals and patients. Nevertheless, a large number of the listed Web sites provide useful background information. We can only recommend this route, therefore, for relatively rare or specific conditions or disorders, or when using highly targeted searches. To use the NIH search utility, visit **http://search.nih.gov/index.html**.

Additional Web Sources

A number of Web sites that often link to government sites are available to the public. These can also point you in the direction of essential information. The following is a representative sample:

- AOL: **http://search.aol.com/cat.adp?id=168&layer=&from=subcats**

- drkoop.com®: **http://www.drkoop.com/conditions/ency/index.html**

- Family Village: **http://www.familyvillage.wisc.edu/specific.htm**

- Google: **http://directory.google.com/Top/Health/Conditions_and_Diseases/**

- Med Help International: **http://www.medhelp.org/HealthTopics/A.html**

- Open Directory Project: **http://dmoz.org/Health/Conditions_and_Diseases/**

- Yahoo.com: **http://dir.yahoo.com/Health/Diseases_and_Conditions/**

- WebMD®Health: **http://my.webmd.com/health_topics**

Vocabulary Builder

The material in this chapter may have contained a number of unfamiliar words. The following Vocabulary Builder introduces you to terms used in this chapter that have not been covered in the previous chapter:

Acromion: The lateral extension of the spine of the scapula and the highest point of the shoulder. [NIH]

Arthroscopy: Endoscopic examination, therapy and surgery of the joint. [NIH]

Bursitis: Inflammation of a bursa, occasionally accompanied by a calcific deposit in the underlying supraspinatus tendon; the most common site is the subdeltoid bursa. [EU]

Cervical: Pertaining to the neck, or to the neck of any organ or structure. [EU]

Chronic: Persisting over a long period of time. [EU]

Degenerative: Undergoing degeneration : tending to degenerate; having the character of or involving degeneration; causing or tending to cause degeneration. [EU]

Dislocation: The displacement of any part, more especially of a bone. Called also luxation. [EU]

Dystocia: Difficult childbirth or labor. [NIH]

Eclampsia: Convulsions and coma occurring in a pregnant or puerperal woman, associated with preeclampsia, i.e., with hypertension, edema, and/or proteinuria. [EU]

Hemorrhage: Bleeding or escape of blood from a vessel. [NIH]

Invasive: 1. having the quality of invasiveness. 2. involving puncture or incision of the skin or insertion of an instrument or foreign material into the body; said of diagnostic techniques. [EU]

Ligament: A band of fibrous tissue that connects bones or cartilages, serving to support and strengthen joints. [EU]

Membrane: A thin layer of tissue which covers a surface, lines a cavity or divides a space or organ. [EU]

Mobility: Capability of movement, of being moved, or of flowing freely. [EU]

Orthopaedic: Pertaining to the correction of deformities of the musculoskeletal system; pertaining to orthopaedics. [EU]

Rheumatology: A subspecialty of internal medicine concerned with the study of inflammatory or degenerative processes and metabolic derangement of connective tissue structures which pertain to a variety of musculoskeletal disorders, such as arthritis. [NIH]

Spondylitis: Inflammation of the vertebrae. [EU]

Surgical: Of, pertaining to, or correctable by surgery. [EU]

Synovial: Of pertaining to, or secreting synovia. [EU]

CHAPTER 2. SEEKING GUIDANCE

Overview

Some patients are comforted by the knowledge that a number of organizations dedicate their resources to helping people with shoulder separation. These associations can become invaluable sources of information and advice. Many associations offer aftercare support, financial assistance, and other important services. Furthermore, healthcare research has shown that support groups often help people to better cope with their conditions.[9] In addition to support groups, your physician can be a valuable source of guidance and support. Therefore, finding a physician that can work with your unique situation is a very important aspect of your care.

In this chapter, we direct you to resources that can help you find patient organizations and medical specialists. We begin by describing how to find associations and peer groups that can help you better understand and cope with shoulder separation. The chapter ends with a discussion on how to find a doctor that is right for you.

Associations and Shoulder Separation

As mentioned by the Agency for Healthcare Research and Quality, sometimes the emotional side of a condition or injury can be as taxing as the physical side.[10] You may have fears or feel overwhelmed by your situation. Everyone has different ways of dealing with disease or physical injury. Your attitude, your expectations, and how well you cope with your condition can

---

[9] Churches, synagogues, and other houses of worship might also have groups that can offer you the social support you need.
[10] This section has been adapted from http://www.ahcpr.gov/consumer/diaginf5.htm.

all influence your well-being. This is true for both minor conditions and serious illnesses. For example, a study on female breast cancer survivors revealed that women who participated in support groups lived longer and experienced better quality of life when compared with women who did not participate. In the support group, women learned coping skills and had the opportunity to share their feelings with other women in the same situation. There are a number of directories that list additional medical associations that you may find useful. While not all of these directories will provide different information, by consulting all of them, you will have nearly exhausted all sources for patient associations.

The National Health Information Center (NHIC)

The National Health Information Center (NHIC) offers a free referral service to help people find organizations that provide information about shoulder separation. For more information, see the NHIC's Web site at **http://www.health.gov/NHIC/** or contact an information specialist by calling 1-800-336-4797.

DIRLINE

A comprehensive source of information on associations is the DIRLINE database maintained by the National Library of Medicine. The database comprises some 10,000 records of organizations, research centers, and government institutes and associations which primarily focus on health and biomedicine. DIRLINE is available via the Internet at the following Web site: **http://dirline.nlm.nih.gov/**. Simply type in "shoulder separation" (or a synonym) or the name of a topic, and the site will list information contained in the database on all relevant organizations.

The Combined Health Information Database

Another comprehensive source of information on healthcare associations is the Combined Health Information Database. Using the "Detailed Search" option, you will need to limit your search to "Organizations" and "shoulder separation". Type the following hyperlink into your Web browser: **http://chid.nih.gov/detail/detail.html**. To find associations, use the drop boxes at the bottom of the search page where "You may refine your search by." For publication date, select "All Years." Then, select your preferred language and the format option "Organization Resource Sheet." By making these selections and typing in "shoulder separation" (or synonyms) into the "For these words:" box, you will only receive results on organizations dealing with shoulder separation. You should check back periodically with this database since it is updated every 3 months.

The National Organization for Rare Disorders, Inc.

The National Organization for Rare Disorders, Inc. has prepared a Web site that provides, at no charge, lists of associations organized by specific conditions and diseases. You can access this database at the following Web site: **http://www.rarediseases.org/cgi-bin/nord/searchpage**. Select the option called "Organizational Database (ODB)" and type "shoulder separation" (or a synonym) in the search box.

Online Support Groups

In addition to support groups, commercial Internet service providers offer forums and chat rooms for people with different illnesses and conditions. WebMD®, for example, offers such a service at their Web site: **http://boards.webmd.com/roundtable**. These online self-help communities can help you connect with a network of people whose concerns are similar to yours. Online support groups are places where people can talk informally. If you read about a novel approach, consult with your doctor or other healthcare providers, as the treatments or discoveries you hear about may not be scientifically proven to be safe and effective.

Finding Doctors

One of the most important aspects of your treatment will be the relationship between you and your doctor or specialist. All patients with shoulder separation must go through the process of selecting a physician. While this process will vary from person to person, the Agency for Healthcare Research and Quality makes a number of suggestions, including the following:[11]

- If you are in a managed care plan, check the plan's list of doctors first.
- Ask doctors or other health professionals who work with doctors, such as hospital nurses, for referrals.

[11] This section is adapted from the AHRQ: www.ahrq.gov/consumer/qntascii/qntdr.htm.

- Call a hospital's doctor referral service, but keep in mind that these services usually refer you to doctors on staff at that particular hospital. The services do not have information on the quality of care that these doctors provide.

- Some local medical societies offer lists of member doctors. Again, these lists do not have information on the quality of care that these doctors provide.

Additional steps you can take to locate doctors include the following:

- Check with the associations listed earlier in this chapter.

- Information on doctors in some states is available on the Internet at **http://www.docboard.org**. This Web site is run by "Administrators in Medicine," a group of state medical board directors.

- The American Board of Medical Specialties can tell you if your doctor is board certified. "Certified" means that the doctor has completed a training program in a specialty and has passed an exam, or "board," to assess his or her knowledge, skills, and experience to provide quality patient care in that specialty. Primary care doctors may also be certified as specialists. The AMBS Web site is located at **http://www.abms.org/newsearch.asp**.[12] You can also contact the ABMS by phone at 1-866-ASK-ABMS.

- You can call the American Medical Association (AMA) at 800-665-2882 for information on training, specialties, and board certification for many licensed doctors in the United States. This information also can be found in "Physician Select" at the AMA's Web site: **http://www.ama-assn.org/aps/amahg.htm**.

If the previous sources did not meet your needs, you may want to log on to the Web site of the National Organization for Rare Disorders (NORD) at **http://www.rarediseases.org/**. NORD maintains a database of doctors with expertise in various rare conditions and diseases. The Metabolic Information Network (MIN), 800-945-2188, also maintains a database of physicians with expertise in various metabolic diseases.

---

[12] While board certification is a good measure of a doctor's knowledge, it is possible to receive quality care from doctors who are not board certified.

Finding an Orthopedic Surgeon

The American Academy of Orthopaedic Surgeons (AAOS) maintains a free-to-use, searchable database of its member doctors. The AAOS members include orthopedic surgeons practicing throughout the U.S. and Canada. To access the database, go to the Academy's home page at **http://www.aaos.org/** and choose "Find a Surgeon" from the menu bar. This will take you to the search form where you can search for member doctors by name or location. To contact the AAOS directly, use the following information:

> **American Academy of Orthopaedic Surgeons**
> P.O. Box 2058
> Des Plaines, IL 60017
> Phone: 800-824-BONE (2663) (free of charge)
> Fax: 847-823-8125
> Fax-on-Demand: 800/999-2939
> **www.aaos.org**

Selecting Your Doctor[3]

When you have compiled a list of prospective doctors, call each of their offices. First, ask if the doctor accepts your health insurance plan and if he or she is taking new patients. If the doctor is not covered by your plan, ask yourself if you are prepared to pay the extra costs. The next step is to schedule a visit with your chosen physician. During the first visit you will have the opportunity to evaluate your doctor and to find out if you feel comfortable with him or her. Ask yourself, did the doctor:

- Give me a chance to ask questions about shoulder separation?

- Really listen to my questions?

- Answer in terms I understood?

- Show respect for me?

- Ask me questions?

- Make me feel comfortable?

- Address the health problem(s) I came with?

- Ask me my preferences about different kinds of treatments for shoulder separation?

---

[13] This section has been adapted from the AHRQ:
www.ahrq.gov/consumer/qntascii/qntdr.htm.

- Spend enough time with me?

Trust your instincts when deciding if the doctor is right for you. But remember, it might take time for the relationship to develop. It takes more than one visit for you and your doctor to get to know each other.

Working with Your Doctor[14]

Research has shown that patients who have good relationships with their doctors tend to be more satisfied with their care and have better results. Here are some tips to help you and your doctor become partners:

- You know important things about your symptoms and your health history. Tell your doctor what you think he or she needs to know.

- It is important to tell your doctor personal information, even if it makes you feel embarrassed or uncomfortable.

- Bring a "health history" list with you (and keep it up to date).

- Always bring any medications you are currently taking with you to the appointment, or you can bring a list of your medications including dosage and frequency information. Talk about any allergies or reactions you have had to your medications.

- Tell your doctor about any natural or alternative medicines you are taking.

- Bring other medical information, such as x-ray films, test results, and medical records.

- Ask questions. If you don't, your doctor will assume that you understood everything that was said.

- Write down your questions before your visit. List the most important ones first to make sure that they are addressed.

- Consider bringing a friend with you to the appointment to help you ask questions. This person can also help you understand and/or remember the answers.

- Ask your doctor to draw pictures if you think that this would help you understand.

- Take notes. Some doctors do not mind if you bring a tape recorder to help you remember things, but always ask first.

---

[14] This section has been adapted from the AHRQ: www.ahrq.gov/consumer/qntascii/qntdr.htm.

- Let your doctor know if you need more time. If there is not time that day, perhaps you can speak to a nurse or physician assistant on staff or schedule a telephone appointment.

- Take information home. Ask for written instructions. Your doctor may also have brochures and audio and videotapes that can help you.

- After leaving the doctor's office, take responsibility for your care. If you have questions, call. If your symptoms get worse or if you have problems with your medication, call. If you had tests and do not hear from your doctor, call for your test results. If your doctor recommended that you have certain tests, schedule an appointment to get them done. If your doctor said you should see an additional specialist, make an appointment.

By following these steps, you will enhance the relationship you will have with your physician.

Broader Health-Related Resources

In addition to the references above, the NIH has set up guidance Web sites that can help patients find healthcare professionals. These include:[15]

- Caregivers:
  http://www.nlm.nih.gov/medlineplus/caregivers.html

- Choosing a Doctor or Healthcare Service:
  http://www.nlm.nih.gov/medlineplus/choosingadoctororhealthcareserv ice.html

- Hospitals and Health Facilities:
  http://www.nlm.nih.gov/medlineplus/healthfacilities.html

---

[15] You can access this information at:
http://www.nlm.nih.gov/medlineplus/healthsystem.html.

PART II: ADDITIONAL RESOURCES AND ADVANCED MATERIAL

ABOUT PART II

In Part II, we introduce you to additional resources and advanced research on shoulder separation. All too often, patients who conduct their own research are overwhelmed by the difficulty in finding and organizing information. The purpose of the following chapters is to provide you an organized and structured format to help you find additional information resources on shoulder separation. In Part II, as in Part I, our objective is not to interpret the latest advances on shoulder separation or render an opinion. Rather, our goal is to give you access to original research and to increase your awareness of sources you may not have already considered. In this way, you will come across the advanced materials often referred to in pamphlets, books, or other general works. Once again, some of this material is technical in nature, so consultation with a professional familiar with shoulder separation is suggested.

CHAPTER 3. STUDIES ON SHOULDER SEPARATION

Overview

Every year, academic studies are published on shoulder separation or related conditions. Broadly speaking, there are two types of studies. The first are peer reviewed. Generally, the content of these studies has been reviewed by scientists or physicians. Peer-reviewed studies are typically published in scientific journals and are usually available at medical libraries. The second type of studies is non-peer reviewed. These works include summary articles that do not use or report scientific results. These often appear in the popular press, newsletters, or similar periodicals.

In this chapter, we will show you how to locate peer-reviewed references and studies on shoulder separation. We will begin by discussing research that has been summarized and is free to view by the public via the Internet. We then show you how to generate a bibliography on shoulder separation and teach you how to keep current on new studies as they are published or undertaken by the scientific community.

The Combined Health Information Database

The Combined Health Information Database summarizes studies across numerous federal agencies. To limit your investigation to research studies and shoulder separation, you will need to use the advanced search options. First, go to **http://chid.nih.gov/index.html**. From there, select the "Detailed Search" option (or go directly to that page with the following hyperlink: **http://chid.nih.gov/detail/detail.html**). The trick in extracting studies is found in the drop boxes at the bottom of the search page where "You may refine your search by." Select the dates and language you prefer, and the format option "Journal Article." At the top of the search form, select the number of records you would like to see (we recommend 100) and check the box to display "whole records." We recommend that you type in "shoulder separation" (or synonyms) into the "For these words:" box. Consider using the option "anywhere in record" to make your search as broad as possible. If you want to limit the search to only a particular field, such as the title of the journal, then select this option in the "Search in these fields" drop box. The following is a sample of what you can expect from this type of search:

- **Painful Shoulder, The: Zeroing in on the Most Common Causes**

  Source: Postgraduate Medicine. 106(7): 36-38,41-43,47-49. December 1999.

  Summary: This journal article provides health professionals with information on the diagnosis and treatment of shoulder pain. Physical examination of the shoulder involves visual inspection, palpation, range of motion testing, strength testing, neurovascular assessment, and general physical evaluation. Diagnostic signs and tests include the Neer impingement sign and the relocation test. Shoulder radiographs are useful in detecting calcification in the capsule or supraspinatus tendon. Magnetic resonance imaging, computed tomography, and other imaging studies may be helpful in reinforcing the physical findings in difficult cases. Shoulder problems that may cause shoulder pain include impingement syndrome, shoulder bursitis, rotator cuff tendinitis, rotator cuff tear, shoulder stiffness, shoulder dislocation and instability, glenohumeral arthritis, acromioclavicular joint problems, shoulder separation, acromioclavicular joint osteoarthritis, and fracture. The article describes these shoulder problems and presents options for treating them. In addition, the article provides information about situations that require referral. 5 figures and 4 references.

The National Library of Medicine: PubMed

One of the quickest and most comprehensive ways to find academic studies in both English and other languages is to use PubMed, maintained by the National Library of Medicine. The advantage of PubMed over previously mentioned sources is that it covers a greater number of domestic and foreign references. It is also free to the public.[16] If the publisher has a Web site that

---

[16] PubMed was developed by the National Center for Biotechnology Information (NCBI) at the National Library of Medicine (NLM) at the National Institutes of Health (NIH). The PubMed database was developed in conjunction with publishers of biomedical literature as a search tool for accessing literature citations and linking to full-text journal articles at Web

offers full text of its journals, PubMed will provide links to that site, as well as to sites offering other related data. User registration, a subscription fee, or some other type of fee may be required to access the full text of articles in some journals.

To generate your own bibliography of studies dealing with shoulder separation, simply go to the PubMed Web site at **www.ncbi.nlm.nih.gov/pubmed**. Type "shoulder separation" (or synonyms) into the search box, and click "Go."

Vocabulary Builder

Calcification: The process by which organic tissue becomes hardened by a deposit of calcium salts within its substance. [EU]

Dysplasia: Abnormality of development; in pathology, alteration in size, shape, and organization of adult cells. [EU]

Hybridization: The genetic process of crossbreeding to produce a hybrid. Hybrid nucleic acids can be formed by nucleic acid hybridization of DNA and RNA molecules. Protein hybridization allows for hybrid proteins to be formed from polypeptide chains. [NIH]

Idiopathic: Of the nature of an idiopathy; self-originated; of unknown causation. [EU]

Lumbar: Pertaining to the loins, the part of the back between the thorax and the pelvis. [EU]

Mineralization: The action of mineralizing; the state of being mineralized. [EU]

Molecular: Of, pertaining to, or composed of molecules : a very small mass of matter. [EU]

Morphogenesis: The development of the form of an organ, part of the body, or organism. [NIH]

Neonatal: Pertaining to the first four weeks after birth. [EU]

Oral: Pertaining to the mouth, taken through or applied in the mouth, as an oral medication or an oral thermometer. [EU]

Osteoarthritis: Noninflammatory degenerative joint disease occurring chiefly in older persons, characterized by degeneration of the articular cartilage, hypertrophy of bone at the margins, and changes in the synovial membrane. It is accompanied by pain and stiffness, particularly after

sites of participating publishers. Publishers that participate in PubMed supply NLM with their citations electronically prior to or at the time of publication.

prolonged activity. [EU]

Palpation: Application of fingers with light pressure to the surface of the body to determine consistence of parts beneath in physical diagnosis; includes palpation for determining the outlines of organs. [NIH]

Phenotype: The outward appearance of the individual. It is the product of interactions between genes and between the genotype and the environment. This includes the killer phenotype, characteristic of yeasts. [NIH]

Radiography: The making of film records (radiographs) of internal structures of the body by passage of x-rays or gamma rays through the body to act on specially sensitized film. [EU]

Tendinitis: Inflammation of tendons and of tendon-muscle attachments. [EU]

Tomography: The recording of internal body images at a predetermined plane by means of the tomograph; called also body section roentgenography. [EU]

CHAPTER 4. BOOKS ON SHOULDER SEPARATION

Overview

This chapter provides bibliographic book references relating to shoulder separation. You have many options to locate books on shoulder separation. The simplest method is to go to your local bookseller and inquire about titles that they have in stock or can special order for you. Some patients, however, feel uncomfortable approaching their local booksellers and prefer online sources (e.g. **www.amazon.com** and **www.bn.com**). In addition to online booksellers, excellent sources for book titles on shoulder separation include the Combined Health Information Database and the National Library of Medicine. Once you have found a title that interests you, visit your local public or medical library to see if it is available for loan.

Book Summaries: Online Booksellers

Commercial Internet-based booksellers, such as Amazon.com and Barnes & Noble.com, offer summaries which have been supplied by each title's publisher. Some summaries also include customer reviews. Your local bookseller may have access to in-house and commercial databases that index all published books (e.g. Books in Print®).

The National Library of Medicine Book Index

The National Library of Medicine at the National Institutes of Health has a massive database of books published on healthcare and biomedicine. Go to the following Internet site, **http://locatorplus.gov/**, and then select "Search LOCATORplus." Once you are in the search area, simply type "shoulder separation" (or synonyms) into the search box, and select "books only." From there, results can be sorted by publication date, author, or relevance. The following was recently catalogued by the National Library of Medicine.[17]

- **Arthroscopy of the upper extremity.**   Author: [edited by] Martti Vastamäki, James H. Roth; Year: 1997; New York: Churchill Livingstone, 1997; ISBN: 0443050015
  http://www.amazon.com/exec/obidos/ASIN/0443050015/icongroupin terna

- **Atlas of shoulder dislocations.**   Author: by H. F. Moseley; illustrations by Helen I. MacArthur; Year: 1951; North Chicago, Ill.: Abbott Laboratories, c1951

- **Atlas of shoulder surgery.**   Author: edited by Freddie H. Fu, Jonathan B. Ticker, Andreas B. Imhoff; with artwork by William R. Filer; Year: 1998; London: Martin Dunitz, 1998; ISBN: 1853172898

- **Atlas of shoulder surgery.**   Author: Richard J. Hawkins, Robert H. Bell, Steven B. Lippitt; illustrated by Larry Howell, Steven B. Lippitt; Year: 1996; St. Louis: Mosby, c1996; ISBN: 0815141963
  http://www.amazon.com/exec/obidos/ASIN/0815141963/icongroupin terna

- **Biomechanics of impact injury and injury tolerances of the thorax-shoulder complex.**   Author: edited by Stanley H. Backaitis; Year: 1994; Warrendale, PA, U.S.A.: Society of Automotive Engineers, c1994; ISBN: 1560915013
  http://www.amazon.com/exec/obidos/ASIN/1560915013/icongroupin terna

- **Clinical challenges in orthopaedics: the shoulder.**   Author: edited by Timothy D. Bunker, Peter J. Schranz; Year: 1998; Oxford: Isis Medical Media; St. Louis, MO, USA: Distributed in the USA by Mosby-Year Book, 1998; ISBN: 1899066748
  http://www.amazon.com/exec/obidos/ASIN/1899066748/icongroupin terna

---

[17] In addition to LOCATORPlus, in collaboration with authors and publishers, the National Center for Biotechnology Information (NCBI) is adapting biomedical books for the Web. The books may be accessed in two ways: (1) by searching directly using any search term or phrase (in the same way as the bibliographic database PubMed), or (2) by following the links to PubMed abstracts. Each PubMed abstract has a "Books" button that displays a facsimile of the abstract in which some phrases are hypertext links. These phrases are also found in the books available at NCBI. Click on hyperlinked results in the list of books in which the phrase is found. Currently, the majority of the links are between the books and PubMed. In the future, more links will be created between the books and other types of information, such as gene and protein sequences and macromolecular structures. See **http://www.ncbi.nlm.nih.gov/entrez/query.fcgi?db=Books.**

- **Complex and revision problems in shoulder surgery.** Author: edited by Jon J.P. Warner, Joseph P. Iannotti, Christian Gerber; 31 contributors; original illustrations by William R. Filer; Year: 1997; Phialdelphia: Lippincott-Raven, c1997; ISBN: 0397516576
http://www.amazon.com/exec/obidos/ASIN/0397516576/icongroupin terna

- **Cuff.** Author: D.F. Gazielly, P. Gleyze, T. Thomas, eds; Year: 1997; Amsterdam; New York: Elsevier, c1997; ISBN: 2906077844
http://www.amazon.com/exec/obidos/ASIN/2906077844/icongroupin terna

- **Diagnosis and treatment of the upper extremities: nonoperative orthopaedic medicine and manual therapy.** Author: Dos Winkel, Omer Matthijs, Valerrie Phelps; Year: 1997; Gaithersburg, Md.: Aspen Publishers, 1997; ISBN: 0834209012
http://www.amazon.com/exec/obidos/ASIN/0834209012/icongroupin terna

- **Disorders of the shoulder: diagnosis and management.** Author: edited by Joseph P. Iannotti, Gerald R. Williams, Jr.; illustrations by Jennifer Smith; Year: 1999; Philadelphia: Lippincott Williams & Wilkins, c1999; ISBN: 078171320X
http://www.amazon.com/exec/obidos/ASIN/078171320X/icongroupi nterna

- **Evaluation and treatment of the shoulder: an integration of the guide to physical therapist practice.** Author: Brian J. Tovin, Bruce H. Greenfield; Year: 2001; Philadelphia: F.A. Davis, c2001; ISBN: 0803602626
http://www.amazon.com/exec/obidos/ASIN/0803602626/icongroupin terna

- **Humerus.** Author: edited by Evan L. Flatow, C. Urich; Year: 1996; Oxford; Boston: Butterworth-Heinemann, 1996; ISBN: 0750608404 (hbk.)
http://www.amazon.com/exec/obidos/ASIN/0750608404/icongroupin terna

- **Joint replacement in the shoulder and elbow.** Author: edited by W. Angus Wallace; Year: 1998; Oxford; Boston: Butterworth-Heinemann, 1998; ISBN: 075061367X
http://www.amazon.com/exec/obidos/ASIN/075061367X/icongroupi nterna

- **Luxations of hip and shoulder.** Author: by Moses Gunn ..; Year: 1855; Ann Arbor: E.B. Pond, Printer ..., 1855

- **Luxations of the hip and shoulder joints, and the agents which oppose their reduction.** Author: by Moses Gunn; Year: 1869; Chicago: Robert Fergus' Sons, Printers ..., 1869

- **Operative shoulder surgery.**   Author: Stephen Copeland; with contributions by Alexander Benjamin, Rolfe Birch; illustrations by Gillian Oliver, Philip Wilson; Year: 1995; New York: Churchill Livingstone, 1995; ISBN: 0443046409
http://www.amazon.com/exec/obidos/ASIN/0443046409/icongroupin terna

- **Orthopaedic knowledge update. Shoulder and elbow.** Author: edited by Tom R. Norris; developed by the American Shoulder and Elbow Surgeons; Year: 1997; Rosemont, IL: American Academy of Orthopaedic Surgeons, c1997; ISBN: 0892031700
http://www.amazon.com/exec/obidos/ASIN/0892031700/icongroupin terna

- **Physical therapy of the shoulder.** Author: edited by Robert A. Donatelli; Year: 1997; New York: Churchill Livingstone, 1997; ISBN: 0443075913 (alk. paper)
http://www.amazon.com/exec/obidos/ASIN/0443075913/icongroupin terna

- **Shoulder: operative technique.**   Author: Melvin Post ... [et al.]; illustrations by Vaune J. Hatch; Year: 1998; Baltimore: Williams & Wilkins, c1998; ISBN: 0683069470
http://www.amazon.com/exec/obidos/ASIN/0683069470/icongroupin terna

- **Shoulder arthroplasty.**   Author: Gilles Walch, Pascal Boileau (eds.); foreword from Norbert Gschwend and Richard J. Hawkins; Year: 1999; Berlin; New York: Springer, c1998; ISBN: 3540633499 (hardcover: alk. paper)
http://www.amazon.com/exec/obidos/ASIN/3540633499/icongroupin terna

- **Shoulder injuries in sport: evaluation, treatment, and rehabilitation.** Author: Jerome Vincent Ciullo; Year: 1996; Champaign, Ill.: Human Kinetics, c1996; ISBN: 0873226518
http://www.amazon.com/exec/obidos/ASIN/0873226518/icongroupin terna

- **Shoulder injuries in the athlete: surgical repair and rehabilitation.** Author: edited by Richard J. Hawkins, Gary W. Misamore; with illustrations by Theodore G. Huff; Year: 1996; New York: Churchill Livingstone, 1996; ISBN: 0443089477
http://www.amazon.com/exec/obidos/ASIN/0443089477/icongroupin terna

- **Shoulder magnetic resonance imaging.** Author: editors, Lynne S. Steinbach ... [et al.]; illustrations by Gilbert M. Gardner; Year: 1998; Philadelphia: Lippincott-Raven, c1998; ISBN: 0397514689 (hc)
  http://www.amazon.com/exec/obidos/ASIN/0397514689/icongroupin terna

- **Shoulder pathophysiology: rehabilitation and treatment.** Author: Scott V. Haig; Year: 1996; Gaithersburg, Md.: Aspen Publishers, 1996; ISBN: 0834206226
  http://www.amazon.com/exec/obidos/ASIN/0834206226/icongroupin terna

- **Shoulder surgery: an illustrated textbook.** Author: edited by Nikolaus Wülker, Michel Mansat, Freddie H. Fu; Year: 2001; London: Martin Dunitz; Malden, MA: Distributed in the U.S. by Blackwell Science, 2001; ISBN: 1853175633
  http://www.amazon.com/exec/obidos/ASIN/1853175633/icongroupin terna

- **Shoulder.** Author: editors, Charles A. Rockwood, Jr., Frederick A. Matsen III; associate editors, Michael A. Wirth, Douglas T. Harryman II; Year: 1998; Philadelphia: Saunders, c1998; ISBN: 0721681344 (set)
  http://www.amazon.com/exec/obidos/ASIN/0721681344/icongroupin terna

- **Surgery of the shoulder: proceedings of the 6th International Congress on Surgery of the Shoulder (ICCS), 27 June-1 July 1995, Helsinki, Finland, and 2-4 July, Stockholm, Sweden.** Author: editors, Martti Vastamäki, Pekka Jalovaara; Year: 1995; Amsterdam; New York: Elsevier, 1995; ISBN: 0444819134 (alk. paper)
  http://www.amazon.com/exec/obidos/ASIN/0444819134/icongroupin terna

- **Unstable shoulder.** Author: editors, Russell F. Warren, Edward V. Craig, David W. Altchek; Year: 1999; Philadelphia: Lippincott-Raven, c1999; ISBN: 0397516770
  http://www.amazon.com/exec/obidos/ASIN/0397516770/icongroupin terna

- **Unstable shoulder.** Author: edited by Louis U. Bigliani; contributors, Robert A. Arciero ... [et al.]; Year: 1996; Rosemont, IL: American Academy of Orthopaedic Surgeons, c1996; ISBN: 0892031204
  http://www.amazon.com/exec/obidos/ASIN/0892031204/icongroupin terna

- **Validation of a human force model to predict dynamic forces resulting from multi-joint motions.** Author: A.K. Pandya ... [et al.]; Year: 1992; Washington, DC: NASA Headquarters, 1992

Chapters on Shoulder Separation

Frequently, shoulder separation will be discussed within a book, perhaps within a specific chapter. In order to find chapters that are specifically dealing with shoulder separation, an excellent source of abstracts is the Combined Health Information Database. You will need to limit your search to book chapters and shoulder separation using the "Detailed Search" option. Go directly to the following hyperlink: **http://chid.nih.gov/detail/detail.html**. To find book chapters, use the drop boxes at the bottom of the search page where "You may refine your search by." Select the dates and language you prefer, and the format option "Book Chapter." By making these selections and typing in "shoulder separation" (or synonyms) into the "For these words:" box, you will only receive results on chapters in books.

General Home References

In addition to references for shoulder separation, you may want a general home medical guide that spans all aspects of home healthcare. The following list is a recent sample of such guides (sorted alphabetically by title; hyperlinks provide rankings, information, and reviews at Amazon.com):

- **American College of Physicians Complete Home Medical Guide (with Interactive Human Anatomy CD-ROM)** by David R. Goldmann (Editor), American College of Physicians; Hardcover - 1104 pages, Book & CD-Rom edition (1999), DK Publishing; ISBN: 0789444127; **http://www.amazon.com/exec/obidos/ASIN/0789444127/icongroupinterna**

- **The American Medical Association Guide to Home Caregiving** by the American Medical Association (Editor); Paperback - 256 pages 1 edition (2001), John Wiley & Sons; ISBN: 0471414093; **http://www.amazon.com/exec/obidos/ASIN/0471414093/icongroupinterna**

- **Anatomica : The Complete Home Medical Reference** by Peter Forrestal (Editor); Hardcover (2000), Book Sales; ISBN: 1740480309; **http://www.amazon.com/exec/obidos/ASIN/1740480309/icongroupinterna**

- **The HarperCollins Illustrated Medical Dictionary : The Complete Home Medical Dictionary** by Ida G. Dox, et al; Paperback - 656 pages 4th edition (2001), Harper Resource; ISBN: 0062736469; **http://www.amazon.com/exec/obidos/ASIN/0062736469/icongroupinterna**

- **Mayo Clinic Guide to Self-Care: Answers for Everyday Health Problems** by Philip Hagen, M.D. (Editor), et al; Paperback - 279 pages, 2nd edition (December 15, 1999), Kensington Publishing Corp.; ISBN: 0962786578; http://www.amazon.com/exec/obidos/ASIN/0962786578/icongroupinterna

- **The Merck Manual of Medical Information : Home Edition (Merck Manual of Medical Information Home Edition (Trade Paper)** by Robert Berkow (Editor), Mark H. Beers, M.D. (Editor); Paperback - 1536 pages (2000), Pocket Books; ISBN: 0671027263; http://www.amazon.com/exec/obidos/ASIN/0671027263/icongroupinterna

Vocabulary Builder

Arthroplasty: Surgical reconstruction of a joint to relieve pain or restore motion. [NIH]

Extremity: A limb; an arm or leg (membrum); sometimes applied specifically to a hand or foot. [EU]

Kinetic: Pertaining to or producing motion. [EU]

Tolerance: 1. the ability to endure unusually large doses of a drug or toxin. 2. acquired drug tolerance; a decreasing response to repeated constant doses of a drug or the need for increasing doses to maintain a constant response. [EU]

CHAPTER 5. MULTIMEDIA ON SHOULDER SEPARATION

Overview

Information on shoulder separation can come in a variety of formats. Among multimedia sources, video productions, slides, audiotapes, and computer databases are often available. In this chapter, we show you how to keep current on multimedia sources of information on shoulder separation. We start with sources that have been summarized by federal agencies, and then show you how to find bibliographic information catalogued by the National Library of Medicine. If you see an interesting item, visit your local medical library to check on the availability of the title.

Bibliography: Multimedia on Shoulder Separation

The National Library of Medicine is a rich source of information on healthcare-related multimedia productions including slides, computer software, and databases. To access the multimedia database, go to the following Web site: **http://locatorplus.gov/**. Select "Search LOCATORplus." Once in the search area, simply type in shoulder separation (or synonyms). Then, in the option box provided below the search box, select "Audiovisuals and Computer Files." From there, you can choose to sort results by publication date, author, or relevance. The following multimedia has been indexed on shoulder separation. For more information, follow the hyperlink indicated:

- **Adhesive strapping in sports for shoulder.** Source: by Duke LaRue; Year: 1999; Format: Videorecording; [Lincoln, Neb.]: R.E. LaRue, c1999

- **Anatomic humeral head replacement.** Source: American Academy of Orthopaedic Surgeons; Year: 1999; Format: Videorecording; Rosemont, Ill.: The Academy, [1999]

- **Anatomy : the shoulder.** Source: a presentation of Films for the Humanities & Sciences; Sheffield University Television; Year: 1999; Format: Videorecording; Princeton, NJ: Films for the Humanities & Sciences, c1999

- **Animated and live techniques of arthroscopic acromioplasty and rotator cuff suture.** Source: the American Academy of Orthopaedic Surgeons; Santa Casa Hospitals, School of Medicine; Year: 2000; Format: Videorecording; Rosemont, Ill.: The Academy, [2000]

- **Anterior Bankart repair : tips on optimizing technique.** Source: the American Academy of Orthopaedic Surgeons; [presented by] United States Navy; production by Medical Media Production Department, Naval School of Health Sciences; Year: 1998; Format: Videorecording; Rosemont, Ill.: The Academy, 1998

- **Anterior capsulolabral reconstruction in the overhead athlete.** Source: the American Academy of Orthopaedic Surgeons, Kerlan-Jobe Orthopaedic Clinic, Centinela Hospital Medical Center; Year: 1999; Format: Videorecording; Rosemont, Ill.: The Academy, [1999]

- **Approach to the shoulder for osteochondritis dissecans.** Source: University of California at Davis, School of Veterinary Medicine; Year: 1978; Format: Videorecording; [Berkeley, Calif.]: Regents of the University of California; [Davis: for loan and sale by University of California, Davis, Health Sciences Television], c1978

- **Arthroscopic anterior shoulder stabilization.** Source: the American Academy of Orthopaedic Surgeons, Kerlan-Jobe Orthopaedic Clinic, Centinela Hospital Medical Center; Year: 1999; Format: Videorecording; Rosemont, Ill.: The Academy, [1999]

- **Arthroscopic Bankart repair with heat probe capsulorrhaphy : double and single anterior cannula techniques.** Source: the American Academy of Orthopaedic Surgeons, Steadman-Hawkins Sports Medicine Foundation; Year: 2000; Format: Videorecording; Rosemont, Ill.: The Academy, [2000]

- **Arthroscopic repair for full-thickness tears of the rotator cuff : surgical technique & outcome analysis.** Source: the American Academy of Orthopaedic Surgeons; a Joe W. King Orthopedic Institute production, in cooperation with Fondren Orthopedi; Year: 1998; Format: Videorecording; Rosemont, Ill.: The Academy, c1998

- **Arthroscopic rotator cuff repair.** Source: the American Academy of Orthopaedic Surgeons; [presented by] Centinela Hospital, in association with Kerlan-Jobe Orthopaedic Center; Year: 1999; Format: Videorecording; Rosemont, Ill.: The Academy, [1999]

- **Basic shoulder arthroscopy and management of the rotator cuff.** Source: [presented by] American Academy of Orthopaedic Surgeons, Southern Sports Medicine & Orthopaedic Center, Baptist Hospital Sports Medicine Center; Year: 2000; Format: Videorecording; Rosemont, Ill.: The Academy, [2000]

- **Biomechanics & injuries of overhand throwing.** Source: ASMT, American Sports Medicine Institute; Year: 2000; Format: Videorecording; Rosemont, Ill.: American Academy of Orthopaedic Surgeons, [2000]

- **C.W. (subpectoral) biceps tenodesis.** Source: the American Academy of Orthopaedic Surgeons; Year: 1999; Format: Videorecording; Rosemont, Ill.: The Academy, [1999]

- **Diagnosis & management of the frozen shoulder.** Source: the American Academy of Orthopaedic Surgeons; [presented by] Centinela Hospital, in association with Kerlan-Jobe Orthopaedic Center; produced by Centinela Hospital's Medical Photography De; Year: 1999; Format: Videorecording; Rosemont, Ill.: The Academy, c1999

- **Diagnosis and surgical management of SLAP lesions.** Source: American Academy of Orthopaedic Surgeons; [presented by] Centinela Hospital, in association with Kerlan-Jobe Orthopaedic Center; Year: 2001; Format: Videorecording; Rosemont, Ill.: The Academy, [2001]

- **Laser capsular shrinkage in the shoulder.** Source: American Academy of Orthopaedic Surgery; Kerlan-Jobe Orthopaedic Clinic; Year: 1998; Format: Videorecording; Rosemont, Ill.: The Academy, [1998]

- **Latissimus dorsi transfer for the treatment of massive rotator cuff tears.** Source: the American Academy of Orthopaedic Surgeons, Steadman-Hawkins Sports Medicine Foundation; Year: 2000; Format: Videorecording; Rosemont, Ill.: The Academy, [2000]

- **Management of 4-part proximal humerus fracture with a prosthesis.** Source: the American Academy of Orthopaedic Surgeons, the University of Texas, Health Science Center at San Antonio; IMS, Information Management & Services; Year: 2000; Format: Videorecording; Rosemont, Ill.: The Academy, c2000

- **New approaches to arthroscopic rotator cuff repair : the subclavian and modified Neviaser portals.** Source: [presented by] American Academy of Orthopaedic Surgeons, West Tennessee Orthopedics & Sports Medicine, Jackson-Madison County General Hosp; Year: 2000; Format: Videorecording; Rosemont, Ill.: The Academy, [2000]

- **Open anterior capsular shift.** Source: American Academy of Orthopaedic Surgeons; produced & presented by ASMI, American Sports

Medicine Institute; Year: 1996; Format: Videorecording; Birmingham, Ala.: American Sports Medicine Institute, c1996

- **Open reduction and lesser tuberosity transfer for acute posterior dislocation of the shoulder.**   Source: the American Academy of Orthopaedic Surgeons, the University of Texas Health Science Center at San Antonio; Year: 1999; Format: Videorecording; Rosemont, Ill.: The Academy, c1999

- **Open reduction and lesser tuberosity transfer for ' acuteposterior dislocation of the shoulder.**   Source: the American Academy of Orthopaedic Surgeons, the University of Texas Health Science Center at San Antonio; Year: 1999; Format: Videorecording; Rosemont, Ill.: The Academy, 1999

- **Peripheral manipulation : a case study in shoulder pain.** Source: G.D. Maitland; Year: 2000; Format: Videorecording; London; Boston: Butterworths, c2000

- **Posterior capsulolabral reconstruction of the shoulder.**   Source: American Academy of Orthopaedic Surgeons; [presented by] Centinela Hospital, in association with Kerlan-Jobe Orthopaedic Center; Year: 1999; Format: Videorecording; Rosemont, Ill.: The Academy, [1999]

- **Revision shoulder arthroplasty.**   Source: American Academy of Orthopaedic Surgeons; the University of Texas Health Science Center at San Antonio; presented by the Department of Orthopaedics, Shoulder Service; produced by the Office of Education; Year: 1997; Format: Videorecording; San Antonio: The University, c1997

- **Shoulder dystocia drill.** Source: the American College of Obstetricians and Gynecologists; Year: 1992; Format: Videorecording; Washington, DC: The College, c1992

- **Surgical approaches to the shoulder.** Source: American Academy of Orthopaedic Surgeons, NYUHJD, NYU, Hospital for Joint Diseases, Department of Orthopaedic Surgery; Year: 2001; Format: Videorecording; Rosemont, Ill.: The Academy, [2001]

- **Surgical management of the impingement syndrome.**   Source: [presented by] Saunders Medical Videos; Year: 1993; Format: Videorecording; Philadelphia: W.B. Saunders, c1993

- **Total shoulder arthroplasty : tips on optimizing technique.** Source: American Academy of Orthopaedic Surgeons; [presented by] United States Navy; production by Medical Media Center; Year: 1997; Format: Videorecording; Rosemont, Ill.: The Academy, 1997

Vocabulary Builder

Cannula: A tube for insertion into a duct or cavity; during insertion its lumen is usually occupied by a trocar. [EU]

Lesion: Any pathological or traumatic discontinuity of tissue or loss of function of a part. [EU]

Orthopedics: A surgical specialty which utilizes medical, surgical, and physical methods to treat and correct deformities, diseases, and injuries to the skeletal system, its articulations, and associated structures. [NIH]

Posterior: Situated in back of, or in the back part of, or affecting the back or dorsal surface of the body. In lower animals, it refers to the caudal end of the body. [EU]

Prosthesis: An artificial substitute for a missing body part, such as an arm or leg, eye or tooth, used for functional or cosmetic reasons, or both. [EU]

Proximal: Nearest; closer to any point of reference; opposed to distal. [EU]

Stabilization: The creation of a stable state. [EU]

PART III. APPENDICES

ABOUT PART III

Part III is a collection of appendices on general medical topics which may be of interest to patients with shoulder separation and related conditions.

APPENDIX A. RESEARCHING YOUR MEDICATIONS

Overview

There are a number of sources available on new or existing medications which could be prescribed to patients with shoulder separation. While a number of hard copy or CD-Rom resources are available to patients and physicians for research purposes, a more flexible method is to use Internet-based databases. In this chapter, we will begin with a general overview of medications. We will then proceed to outline official recommendations on how you should view your medications. You may also want to research medications that you are currently taking for other conditions as they may interact with medications for shoulder separation. Research can give you information on the side effects, interactions, and limitations of prescription drugs used in the treatment of shoulder separation. Broadly speaking, there are two sources of information on approved medications: public sources and private sources. We will emphasize free-to-use public sources.

Your Medications: The Basics[18]

The Agency for Health Care Research and Quality has published extremely useful guidelines on how you can best participate in the medication aspects of shoulder separation. Taking medicines is not always as simple as swallowing a pill. It can involve many steps and decisions each day. The AHCRQ recommends that patients with shoulder separation take part in treatment decisions. Do not be afraid to ask questions and talk about your concerns. By taking a moment to ask questions early, you may avoid problems later. Here are some points to cover each time a new medicine is prescribed:

- Ask about all parts of your treatment, including diet changes, exercise, and medicines.

- Ask about the risks and benefits of each medicine or other treatment you might receive.

- Ask how often you or your doctor will check for side effects from a given medication.

Do not hesitate to ask what is important to you about your medicines. You may want a medicine with the fewest side effects, or the fewest doses to take each day. You may care most about cost, or how the medicine might affect how you live or work. Or, you may want the medicine your doctor believes will work the best. Telling your doctor will help him or her select the best treatment for you.

Do not be afraid to "bother" your doctor with your concerns and questions about medications for shoulder separation. You can also talk to a nurse or a pharmacist. They can help you better understand your treatment plan. Feel free to bring a friend or family member with you when you visit your doctor. Talking over your options with someone you trust can help you make better choices, especially if you are not feeling well. Specifically, ask your doctor the following:

- The name of the medicine and what it is supposed to do.

- How and when to take the medicine, how much to take, and for how long.

- What food, drinks, other medicines, or activities you should avoid while taking the medicine.

- What side effects the medicine may have, and what to do if they occur.

---

[18] This section is adapted from AHCRQ: **http://www.ahcpr.gov/consumer/ncpiebro.htm** .

- If you can get a refill, and how often.

- About any terms or directions you do not understand.

- What to do if you miss a dose.

- If there is written information you can take home (most pharmacies have information sheets on your prescription medicines; some even offer large-print or Spanish versions).

Do not forget to tell your doctor about all the medicines you are currently taking (not just those for shoulder separation). This includes prescription medicines and the medicines that you buy over the counter. Then your doctor can avoid giving you a new medicine that may not work well with the medications you take now. When talking to your doctor, you may wish to prepare a list of medicines you currently take, the reason you take them, and how you take them. Be sure to include the following information for each:

- Name of medicine

- Reason taken

- Dosage

- Time(s) of day

Also include any over-the-counter medicines, such as:

- Laxatives

- Diet pills

- Vitamins

- Cold medicine

- Aspirin or other pain, headache, or fever medicine

- Cough medicine

- Allergy relief medicine

- Antacids

- Sleeping pills

- Others (include names)

Learning More about Your Medications

Because of historical investments by various organizations and the emergence of the Internet, it has become rather simple to learn about the medications your doctor has recommended for shoulder separation. One such source is the United States Pharmacopeia. In 1820, eleven physicians met in Washington, D.C. to establish the first compendium of standard drugs for the United States. They called this compendium the "U.S. Pharmacopeia (USP)." Today, the USP is a non-profit organization consisting of 800 volunteer scientists, eleven elected officials, and 400 representatives of state associations and colleges of medicine and pharmacy. The USP is located in Rockville, Maryland, and its home page is located at **www.usp.org**. The USP currently provides standards for over 3,700 medications. The resulting USP DI® Advice for the Patient® can be accessed through the National Library of Medicine of the National Institutes of Health. The database is partially derived from lists of federally approved medications in the Food and Drug Administration's (FDA) Drug Approvals database.[19]

While the FDA database is rather large and difficult to navigate, the Phamacopeia is both user-friendly and free to use. It covers more than 9,000 prescription and over-the-counter medications. To access this database, simply type the following hyperlink into your Web browser: **http://www.nlm.nih.gov/medlineplus/druginformation.html**. To view examples of a given medication (brand names, category, description, preparation, proper use, precautions, side effects, etc.), simply follow the hyperlinks indicated within the United States Pharmacopoeia (USP). It is important to read the disclaimer by the USP (**http://www.nlm.nih.gov/medlineplus/drugdisclaimer.html**) before using the information provided.

Commercial Databases

In addition to the medications listed in the USP above, a number of commercial sites are available by subscription to physicians and their institutions. You may be able to access these sources from your local medical library or your doctor's office.

---

[19] Though cumbersome, the FDA database can be freely browsed at the following site: **www.fda.gov/cder/da/da.htm**.

Reuters Health Drug Database

The Reuters Health Drug Database can be searched by keyword at the hyperlink: **http://www.reutershealth.com/frame2/drug.html**.

Mosby's GenRx

Mosby's GenRx database (also available on CD-Rom and book format) covers 45,000 drug products including generics and international brands. It provides prescribing information, drug interactions, and patient information. Information in Mosby's GenRx database can be obtained at the following hyperlink: **http://www.genrx.com/Mosby/PhyGenRx/group.html**.

Physicians Desk Reference

The Physicians Desk Reference database (also available in CD-Rom and book format) is a full-text drug database. The database is searchable by brand name, generic name or by indication. It features multiple drug interactions reports. Information can be obtained at the following hyperlink: **http://physician.pdr.net/physician/templates/en/acl/psuser_t.htm**.

Other Web Sites

A number of additional Web sites discuss drug information. As an example, you may like to look at **www.drugs.com** which reproduces the information in the Pharmacopeia as well as commercial information. You may also want to consider the Web site of the Medical Letter, Inc. which allows users to download articles on various drugs and therapeutics for a nominal fee: **http://www.medletter.com/**.

Contraindications and Interactions (Hidden Dangers)

Some of the medications mentioned in the previous discussions can be problematic for patients with shoulder separation--not because they are used in the treatment process, but because of contraindications, or side effects. Medications with contraindications are those that could react with drugs used to treat shoulder separation or potentially create deleterious side effects in patients with shoulder separation. You should ask your physician about any contraindications, especially as these might apply to other medications that you may be taking for common ailments.

Drug-drug interactions occur when two or more drugs react with each other. This drug-drug interaction may cause you to experience an unexpected side effect. Drug interactions may make your medications less effective, cause unexpected side effects, or increase the action of a particular drug. Some drug interactions can even be harmful to you.

Be sure to read the label every time you use a nonprescription or prescription drug, and take the time to learn about drug interactions. These precautions may be critical to your health. You can reduce the risk of potentially harmful drug interactions and side effects with a little bit of knowledge and common sense.

Drug labels contain important information about ingredients, uses, warnings, and directions which you should take the time to read and understand. Labels also include warnings about possible drug interactions. Further, drug labels may change as new information becomes available. This is why it's especially important to read the label every time you use a medication. When your doctor prescribes a new drug, discuss all over-the-counter and prescription medications, dietary supplements, vitamins, botanicals, minerals and herbals you take as well as the foods you eat. Ask your pharmacist for the package insert for each prescription drug you take. The package insert provides more information about potential drug interactions.

A Final Warning

At some point, you may hear of alternative medications from friends, relatives, or in the news media. Advertisements may suggest that certain alternative drugs can produce positive results for patients with shoulder separation. Exercise caution--some of these drugs may have fraudulent claims, and others may actually hurt you. The Food and Drug Administration (FDA) is the official U.S. agency charged with discovering which medications are likely to improve the health of patients with shoulder separation. The FDA warns patients to watch out for[20]:

- Secret formulas (real scientists share what they know)

---

[20] This section has been adapted from
http://www.fda.gov/opacom/lowlit/medfraud.html.

- Amazing breakthroughs or miracle cures (real breakthroughs don't happen very often; when they do, real scientists do not call them amazing or miracles)

- Quick, painless, or guaranteed cures

- If it sounds too good to be true, it probably isn't true.

If you have any questions about any kind of medical treatment, the FDA may have an office near you. Look for their number in the blue pages of the phone book. You can also contact the FDA through its toll-free number, 1-888-INFO-FDA (1-888-463-6332), or on the World Wide Web at **www.fda.gov**.

General References

In addition to the resources provided earlier in this chapter, the following general references describe medications (sorted alphabetically by title; hyperlinks provide rankings, information and reviews at Amazon.com):

- **Complete Guide to Prescription and Nonprescription Drugs 2001 (Complete Guide to Prescription and Nonprescription Drugs, 2001)** by H. Winter Griffith, Paperback 16th edition (2001), Medical Surveillance; ISBN: 0942447417;
http://www.amazon.com/exec/obidos/ASIN/039952634X/icongroupinterna

- **The Essential Guide to Prescription Drugs, 2001** by James J. Rybacki, James W. Long; Paperback - 1274 pages (2001), Harper Resource; ISBN: 0060958162;
http://www.amazon.com/exec/obidos/ASIN/0060958162/icongroupinterna

- **Handbook of Commonly Prescribed Drugs** by G. John Digregorio, Edward J. Barbieri; Paperback 16th edition (2001), Medical Surveillance; ISBN: 0942447417;
http://www.amazon.com/exec/obidos/ASIN/0942447417/icongroupinterna

- **Johns Hopkins Complete Home Encyclopedia of Drugs 2nd ed.** by Simeon Margolis (Ed.), Johns Hopkins; Hardcover - 835 pages (2000), Rebus; ISBN: 0929661583;
http://www.amazon.com/exec/obidos/ASIN/0929661583/icongroupinterna

- **Medical Pocket Reference: Drugs 2002** by Springhouse Paperback 1st edition (2001), Lippincott Williams & Wilkins Publishers; ISBN: 1582550964;
http://www.amazon.com/exec/obidos/ASIN/1582550964/icongroupinterna

- **PDR** by Medical Economics Staff, Medical Economics Staff Hardcover - 3506 pages 55th edition (2000), Medical Economics Company; ISBN: 1563633752;
http://www.amazon.com/exec/obidos/ASIN/1563633752/icongroupinterna

- **Pharmacy Simplified: A Glossary of Terms** by James Grogan; Paperback - 432 pages, 1st edition (2001), Delmar Publishers; ISBN: 0766828581;
http://www.amazon.com/exec/obidos/ASIN/0766828581/icongroupinterna

- **Physician Federal Desk Reference** by Christine B. Fraizer; Paperback 2nd edition (2001), Medicode Inc; ISBN: 1563373971;
http://www.amazon.com/exec/obidos/ASIN/1563373971/icongroupinterna

- **Physician's Desk Reference Supplements** Paperback - 300 pages, 53 edition (1999), ISBN: 1563632950;
http://www.amazon.com/exec/obidos/ASIN/1563632950/icongroupinterna

APPENDIX B. RESEARCHING NUTRITION

Overview

Since the time of Hippocrates, doctors have understood the importance of diet and nutrition to patients' health and well-being. Since then, they have accumulated an impressive archive of studies and knowledge dedicated to this subject. Based on their experience, doctors and healthcare providers may recommend particular dietary supplements to patients with shoulder separation. Any dietary recommendation is based on a patient's age, body mass, gender, lifestyle, eating habits, food preferences, and health condition. It is therefore likely that different patients with shoulder separation may be given different recommendations. Some recommendations may be directly related to shoulder separation, while others may be more related to the patient's general health. These recommendations, themselves, may differ from what official sources recommend for the average person.

In this chapter we will begin by briefly reviewing the essentials of diet and nutrition that will broadly frame more detailed discussions of shoulder separation. We will then show you how to find studies dedicated specifically to nutrition and shoulder separation.

Food and Nutrition: General Principles

What Are Essential Foods?

Food is generally viewed by official sources as consisting of six basic elements: (1) fluids, (2) carbohydrates, (3) protein, (4) fats, (5) vitamins, and (6) minerals. Consuming a combination of these elements is considered to be a healthy diet:

- **Fluids** are essential to human life as 80-percent of the body is composed of water. Water is lost via urination, sweating, diarrhea, vomiting, diuretics (drugs that increase urination), caffeine, and physical exertion.

- **Carbohydrates** are the main source for human energy (thermoregulation) and the bulk of typical diets. They are mostly classified as being either simple or complex. Simple carbohydrates include sugars which are often consumed in the form of cookies, candies, or cakes. Complex carbohydrates consist of starches and dietary fibers. Starches are consumed in the form of pastas, breads, potatoes, rice, and other foods. Soluble fibers can be eaten in the form of certain vegetables, fruits, oats, and legumes. Insoluble fibers include brown rice, whole grains, certain fruits, wheat bran and legumes.

- **Proteins** are eaten to build and repair human tissues. Some foods that are high in protein are also high in fat and calories. Food sources for protein include nuts, meat, fish, cheese, and other dairy products.

- **Fats** are consumed for both energy and the absorption of certain vitamins. There are many types of fats, with many general publications recommending the intake of unsaturated fats or those low in cholesterol.

Vitamins and minerals are fundamental to human health, growth, and, in some cases, disease prevention. Most are consumed in your diet (exceptions being vitamins K and D which are produced by intestinal bacteria and sunlight on the skin, respectively). Each vitamin and mineral plays a different role in health. The following outlines essential vitamins:

- **Vitamin A** is important to the health of your eyes, hair, bones, and skin; sources of vitamin A include foods such as eggs, carrots, and cantaloupe.

- **Vitamin B^1**, also known as thiamine, is important for your nervous system and energy production; food sources for thiamine include meat, peas, fortified cereals, bread, and whole grains.

- **Vitamin B^2**, also known as riboflavin, is important for your nervous system and muscles, but is also involved in the release of proteins from nutrients; food sources for riboflavin include dairy products, leafy vegetables, meat, and eggs.

- **Vitamin B^3**, also known as niacin, is important for healthy skin and helps the body use energy; food sources for niacin include peas, peanuts, fish, and whole grains

- **Vitamin B^6**, also known as pyridoxine, is important for the regulation of cells in the nervous system and is vital for blood formation; food sources for pyridoxine include bananas, whole grains, meat, and fish.

- **Vitamin B^{12}** is vital for a healthy nervous system and for the growth of red blood cells in bone marrow; food sources for vitamin B^{12} include yeast, milk, fish, eggs, and meat.

- **Vitamin C** allows the body's immune system to fight various diseases, strengthens body tissue, and improves the body's use of iron; food sources for vitamin C include a wide variety of fruits and vegetables.

- **Vitamin D** helps the body absorb calcium which strengthens bones and teeth; food sources for vitamin D include oily fish and dairy products.

- **Vitamin E** can help protect certain organs and tissues from various degenerative diseases; food sources for vitamin E include margarine, vegetables, eggs, and fish.

- **Vitamin K** is essential for bone formation and blood clotting; common food sources for vitamin K include leafy green vegetables.

- **Folic Acid** maintains healthy cells and blood and, when taken by a pregnant woman, can prevent her fetus from developing neural tube defects; food sources for folic acid include nuts, fortified breads, leafy green vegetables, and whole grains.

It should be noted that one can overdose on certain vitamins which become toxic if consumed in excess (e.g. vitamin A, D, E and K).

Like vitamins, minerals are chemicals that are required by the body to remain in good health. Because the human body does not manufacture these chemicals internally, we obtain them from food and other dietary sources. The more important minerals include:

- **Calcium** is needed for healthy bones, teeth, and muscles, but also helps the nervous system function; food sources for calcium include dry beans, peas, eggs, and dairy products.

- **Chromium** is helpful in regulating sugar levels in blood; food sources for chromium include egg yolks, raw sugar, cheese, nuts, beets, whole grains, and meat.

- **Fluoride** is used by the body to help prevent tooth decay and to reinforce bone strength; sources of fluoride include drinking water and certain brands of toothpaste.

- **Iodine** helps regulate the body's use of energy by synthesizing into the hormone thyroxine; food sources include leafy green vegetables, nuts, egg yolks, and red meat.

- **Iron** helps maintain muscles and the formation of red blood cells and certain proteins; food sources for iron include meat, dairy products, eggs, and leafy green vegetables.

- **Magnesium** is important for the production of DNA, as well as for healthy teeth, bones, muscles, and nerves; food sources for magnesium include dried fruit, dark green vegetables, nuts, and seafood.

- **Phosphorous** is used by the body to work with calcium to form bones and teeth; food sources for phosphorous include eggs, meat, cereals, and dairy products.

- **Selenium** primarily helps maintain normal heart and liver functions; food sources for selenium include wholegrain cereals, fish, meat, and dairy products.

- **Zinc** helps wounds heal, the formation of sperm, and encourage rapid growth and energy; food sources include dried beans, shellfish, eggs, and nuts.

The United States government periodically publishes recommended diets and consumption levels of the various elements of food. Again, your doctor may encourage deviations from the average official recommendation based on your specific condition. To learn more about basic dietary guidelines, visit the Web site: **http://www.health.gov/dietaryguidelines/**. Based on these guidelines, many foods are required to list the nutrition levels on the food's packaging. Labeling Requirements are listed at the following site maintained by the Food and Drug Administration: **http://www.cfsan.fda.gov/~dms/lab-cons.html**. When interpreting these requirements, the government recommends that consumers become familiar with the following abbreviations before reading FDA literature:[21]

- **DVs (Daily Values):** A new dietary reference term that will appear on the food label. It is made up of two sets of references, DRVs and RDIs.

- **DRVs (Daily Reference Values):** A set of dietary references that applies to fat, saturated fat, cholesterol, carbohydrate, protein, fiber, sodium, and potassium.

---

[21] Adapted from the FDA: **http://www.fda.gov/fdac/special/foodlabel/dvs.html**.

- **RDIs (Reference Daily Intakes):** A set of dietary references based on the Recommended Dietary Allowances for essential vitamins and minerals and, in selected groups, protein. The name "RDI" replaces the term "U.S. RDA."

- **RDAs (Recommended Dietary Allowances):** A set of estimated nutrient allowances established by the National Academy of Sciences. It is updated periodically to reflect current scientific knowledge.

What Are Dietary Supplements?[22]

Dietary supplements are widely available through many commercial sources, including health food stores, grocery stores, pharmacies, and by mail. Dietary supplements are provided in many forms including tablets, capsules, powders, gel-tabs, extracts, and liquids. Historically in the United States, the most prevalent type of dietary supplement was a multivitamin/mineral tablet or capsule that was available in pharmacies, either by prescription or "over the counter." Supplements containing strictly herbal preparations were less widely available. Currently in the United States, a wide array of supplement products are available, including vitamin, mineral, other nutrients, and botanical supplements as well as ingredients and extracts of animal and plant origin.

The Office of Dietary Supplements (ODS) of the National Institutes of Health is the official agency of the United States which has the expressed goal of acquiring "new knowledge to help prevent, detect, diagnose, and treat disease and disability, from the rarest genetic disorder to the common cold."[23] According to the ODS, dietary supplements can have an important impact on the prevention and management of disease and on the maintenance of health.[24] The ODS notes that considerable research on the effects of dietary supplements has been conducted in Asia and Europe where the use of plant products, in particular, has a long tradition. However, the

---

[22] This discussion has been adapted from the NIH:
http://ods.od.nih.gov/whatare/whatare.html.

[23] Contact: The Office of Dietary Supplements, National Institutes of Health, Building 31, Room 1B29, 31 Center Drive, MSC 2086, Bethesda, Maryland 20892-2086, Tel: (301) 435-2920, Fax: (301) 480-1845, E-mail: **ods@nih.gov**.

[24] Adapted from **http://ods.od.nih.gov/about/about.html**. The Dietary Supplement Health and Education Act defines dietary supplements as "a product (other than tobacco) intended to supplement the diet that bears or contains one or more of the following dietary ingredients: a vitamin, mineral, amino acid, herb or other botanical; or a dietary substance for use to supplement the diet by increasing the total dietary intake; or a concentrate, metabolite, constituent, extract, or combination of any ingredient described above; and intended for ingestion in the form of a capsule, powder, softgel, or gelcap, and not represented as a conventional food or as a sole item of a meal or the diet."

overwhelming majority of supplements have not been studied scientifically. To explore the role of dietary supplements in the improvement of health care, the ODS plans, organizes, and supports conferences, workshops, and symposia on scientific topics related to dietary supplements. The ODS often works in conjunction with other NIH Institutes and Centers, other government agencies, professional organizations, and public advocacy groups.

To learn more about official information on dietary supplements, visit the ODS site at **http://ods.od.nih.gov/whatare/whatare.html**. Or contact:

> The Office of Dietary Supplements
> National Institutes of Health
> Building 31, Room 1B29
> 31 Center Drive, MSC 2086
> Bethesda, Maryland 20892-2086
> Tel: (301) 435-2920
> Fax: (301) 480-1845
> E-mail: ods@nih.gov

Finding Studies on Shoulder Separation

The NIH maintains an office dedicated to patient nutrition and diet. The National Institutes of Health's Office of Dietary Supplements (ODS) offers a searchable bibliographic database called the IBIDS (International Bibliographic Information on Dietary Supplements). The IBIDS contains over 460,000 scientific citations and summaries about dietary supplements and nutrition as well as references to published international, scientific literature on dietary supplements such as vitamins, minerals, and botanicals.[25] IBIDS is available to the public free of charge through the ODS Internet page: **http://ods.od.nih.gov/databases/ibids.html**.

After entering the search area, you have three choices: (1) IBIDS Consumer Database, (2) Full IBIDS Database, or (3) Peer Reviewed Citations Only. We recommend that you start with the Consumer Database. While you may not find references for the topics that are of most interest to you, check back periodically as this database is frequently updated. More studies can be

---

[25] Adapted from http://ods.od.nih.gov. IBIDS is produced by the Office of Dietary Supplements (ODS) at the National Institutes of Health to assist the public, healthcare providers, educators, and researchers in locating credible, scientific information on dietary supplements. IBIDS was developed and will be maintained through an interagency partnership with the Food and Nutrition Information Center of the National Agricultural Library, U.S. Department of Agriculture.

found by searching the Full IBIDS Database. Healthcare professionals and researchers generally use the third option, which lists peer-reviewed citations. In all cases, we suggest that you take advantage of the "Advanced Search" option that allows you to retrieve up to 100 fully explained references in a comprehensive format. Type "shoulder separation" (or synonyms) into the search box. To narrow the search, you can also select the "Title" field.

The following information is typical of that found when using the "Full IBIDS Database" when searching using "shoulder separation" (or a synonym):

- **Effect of dietary selenium source, level, and pig hair color on various selenium indices.**
  Author(s): Department of Animal Sciences, The Ohio State University and The Ohio Agricultural Research and Development Center, Columbus 43210, USA.
  Source: Kim, Y Y Mahan, D C J-Anim-Sci. 2001 April; 79(4): 949-55 0021-8812

- **Frequency of fractures in women with systemic lupus erythematosus: comparison with United States population data.**
  Author(s): Northwestern University, Chicago, Illinois, USA.
  Source: Ramsey Goldman, R Dunn, J E Huang, C F Dunlop, D Rairie, J E Fitzgerald, S Manzi, S Arthritis-Rheum. 1999 May; 42(5): 882-90 0004-3591

- **Metabolic fate of partially depolymerized chondroitin sulfate administered to the rat.**
  Author(s): Institute of Biological Chemistry, School of Medicine, University of Pisa, Italy.
  Source: Conte, A Palmieri, L Segnini, D Ronca, G Drugs-Exp-Clin-Res. 1991; 17(1): 27-33 0378-6501

Federal Resources on Nutrition

In addition to the IBIDS, the United States Department of Health and Human Services (HHS) and the United States Department of Agriculture (USDA) provide many sources of information on general nutrition and health. Recommended resources include:

- healthfinder®, HHS's gateway to health information, including diet and nutrition:
  http://www.healthfinder.gov/scripts/SearchContext.asp?topic=238&page=0

- The United States Department of Agriculture's Web site dedicated to nutrition information: **www.nutrition.gov**

- The Food and Drug Administration's Web site for federal food safety information: **www.foodsafety.gov**

- The National Action Plan on Overweight and Obesity sponsored by the United States Surgeon General: **http://www.surgeongeneral.gov/topics/obesity/**

- The Center for Food Safety and Applied Nutrition has an Internet site sponsored by the Food and Drug Administration and the Department of Health and Human Services: **http://vm.cfsan.fda.gov/**

- Center for Nutrition Policy and Promotion sponsored by the United States Department of Agriculture: **http://www.usda.gov/cnpp/**

- Food and Nutrition Information Center, National Agricultural Library sponsored by the United States Department of Agriculture: **http://www.nal.usda.gov/fnic/**

- Food and Nutrition Service sponsored by the United States Department of Agriculture: **http://www.fns.usda.gov/fns/**

Additional Web Resources

A number of additional Web sites offer encyclopedic information covering food and nutrition. The following is a representative sample:

- AOL: **http://search.aol.com/cat.adp?id=174&layer=&from=subcats**

- Family Village: **http://www.familyvillage.wisc.edu/med_nutrition.html**

- Google: **http://directory.google.com/Top/Health/Nutrition/**

- Healthnotes: **http://www.thedacare.org/healthnotes/**

- Open Directory Project: **http://dmoz.org/Health/Nutrition/**

- Yahoo.com: **http://dir.yahoo.com/Health/Nutrition/**

- WebMD®Health: **http://my.webmd.com/nutrition**

- WholeHealthMD.com: **http://www.wholehealthmd.com/reflib/0,1529,,00.html**

Vocabulary Builder

The following vocabulary builder defines words used in the references in this chapter that have not been defined in previous chapters:

Bacteria: Unicellular prokaryotic microorganisms which generally possess rigid cell walls, multiply by cell division, and exhibit three principal forms: round or coccal, rodlike or bacillary, and spiral or spirochetal. [NIH]

Capsules: Hard or soft soluble containers used for the oral administration of medicine. [NIH]

Carbohydrate: An aldehyde or ketone derivative of a polyhydric alcohol, particularly of the pentahydric and hexahydric alcohols. They are so named because the hydrogen and oxygen are usually in the proportion to form water, $(CH_2O)n$. The most important carbohydrates are the starches, sugars, celluloses, and gums. They are classified into mono-, di-, tri-, poly- and heterosaccharides. [EU]

Cholesterol: The principal sterol of all higher animals, distributed in body tissues, especially the brain and spinal cord, and in animal fats and oils. [NIH]

Diarrhea: Passage of excessively liquid or excessively frequent stools. [NIH]

Intestinal: Pertaining to the intestine. [EU]

Iodine: A nonmetallic element of the halogen group that is represented by the atomic symbol I, atomic number 53, and atomic weight of 126.90. It is a nutritionally essential element, especially important in thyroid hormone synthesis. In solution, it has anti-infective properties and is used topically. [NIH]

Lupus: A form of cutaneous tuberculosis. It is seen predominantly in women and typically involves the nasal, buccal, and conjunctival mucosa. [NIH]

Neural: 1. pertaining to a nerve or to the nerves. 2. situated in the region of the spinal axis, as the neutral arch. [EU]

Niacin: Water-soluble vitamin of the B complex occurring in various animal and plant tissues. Required by the body for the formation of coenzymes NAD and NADP. Has pellagra-curative, vasodilating, and antilipemic properties. [NIH]

Overdose: 1. to administer an excessive dose. 2. an excessive dose. [EU]

Potassium: An element that is in the alkali group of metals. It has an atomic symbol K, atomic number 19, and atomic weight 39.10. It is the chief cation in the intracellular fluid of muscle and other cells. Potassium ion is a strong electrolyte and it plays a significant role in the regulation of fluid volume and maintenance of the water-electrolyte balance. [NIH]

Proteins: Polymers of amino acids linked by peptide bonds. The specific sequence of amino acids determines the shape and function of the protein. [NIH]

Riboflavin: Nutritional factor found in milk, eggs, malted barley, liver, kidney, heart, and leafy vegetables. The richest natural source is yeast. It occurs in the free form only in the retina of the eye, in whey, and in urine; its principal forms in tissues and cells are as FMN and FAD. [NIH]

Selenium: An element with the atomic symbol Se, atomic number 34, and atomic weight 78.96. It is an essential micronutrient for mammals and other animals but is toxic in large amounts. Selenium protects intracellular structures against oxidative damage. It is an essential component of glutathione peroxidase. [NIH]

Systemic: Pertaining to or affecting the body as a whole. [EU]

Thermoregulation: Heat regulation. [EU]

Thyroxine: An amino acid of the thyroid gland which exerts a stimulating effect on thyroid metabolism. [NIH]

Toxic: Pertaining to, due to, or of the nature of a poison or toxin; manifesting the symptoms of severe infection. [EU]

APPENDIX C. FINDING MEDICAL LIBRARIES

Overview

At a medical library you can find medical texts and reference books, consumer health publications, specialty newspapers and magazines, as well as medical journals. In this Appendix, we show you how to quickly find a medical library in your area.

Preparation

Before going to the library, highlight the references mentioned in this sourcebook that you find interesting. Focus on those items that are not available via the Internet, and ask the reference librarian for help with your search. He or she may know of additional resources that could be helpful to you. Most importantly, your local public library and medical libraries have Interlibrary Loan programs with the National Library of Medicine (NLM), one of the largest medical collections in the world. According to the NLM, most of the literature in the general and historical collections of the National Library of Medicine is available on interlibrary loan to any library. NLM's interlibrary loan services are only available to libraries. If you would like to access NLM medical literature, then visit a library in your area that can request the publications for you.[26]

---

[26] Adapted from the NLM: http://www.nlm.nih.gov/psd/cas/interlibrary.html.

Finding a Local Medical Library

The quickest method to locate medical libraries is to use the Internet-based directory published by the National Network of Libraries of Medicine (NN/LM). This network includes 4626 members and affiliates that provide many services to librarians, health professionals, and the public. To find a library in your area, simply visit **http://nnlm.gov/members/adv.html** or call 1-800-338-7657.

Medical Libraries Open to the Public

In addition to the NN/LM, the National Library of Medicine (NLM) lists a number of libraries that are generally open to the public and have reference facilities. The following is the NLM's list plus hyperlinks to each library Web site. These Web pages can provide information on hours of operation and other restrictions. The list below is a small sample of libraries recommended by the National Library of Medicine (sorted alphabetically by name of the U.S. state or Canadian province where the library is located):[27]

- **Alabama:** Health InfoNet of Jefferson County (Jefferson County Library Cooperative, Lister Hill Library of the Health Sciences), **http://www.uab.edu/infonet/**

- **Alabama:** Richard M. Scrushy Library (American Sports Medicine Institute), **http://www.asmi.org/LIBRARY.HTM**

- **Arizona:** Samaritan Regional Medical Center: The Learning Center (Samaritan Health System, Phoenix, Arizona), **http://www.samaritan.edu/library/bannerlibs.htm**

- **California:** Kris Kelly Health Information Center (St. Joseph Health System), **http://www.humboldt1.com/~kkhic/index.html**

- **California:** Community Health Library of Los Gatos (Community Health Library of Los Gatos), **http://www.healthlib.org/orgresources.html**

- **California:** Consumer Health Program and Services (CHIPS) (County of Los Angeles Public Library, Los Angeles County Harbor-UCLA Medical Center Library) - Carson, CA, **http://www.colapublib.org/services/chips.html**

- **California:** Gateway Health Library (Sutter Gould Medical Foundation)

- **California:** Health Library (Stanford University Medical Center), **http://www-med.stanford.edu/healthlibrary/**

---

[27] Abstracted from **http://www.nlm.nih.gov/medlineplus/libraries.html**

- **California:** Patient Education Resource Center - Health Information and Resources (University of California, San Francisco), **http://sfghdean.ucsf.edu/barnett/PERC/default.asp**

- **California:** Redwood Health Library (Petaluma Health Care District), **http://www.phcd.org/rdwdlib.html**

- **California:** San José PlaneTree Health Library, **http://planetreesanjose.org/**

- **California:** Sutter Resource Library (Sutter Hospitals Foundation), **http://go.sutterhealth.org/comm/resc-library/sac-resources.html**

- **California:** University of California, Davis. Health Sciences Libraries

- **California:** ValleyCare Health Library & Ryan Comer Cancer Resource Center (ValleyCare Health System), **http://www.valleycare.com/library.html**

- **California:** Washington Community Health Resource Library (Washington Community Health Resource Library), **http://www.healthlibrary.org/**

- **Colorado:** William V. Gervasini Memorial Library (Exempla Healthcare), **http://www.exempla.org/conslib.htm**

- **Connecticut:** Hartford Hospital Health Science Libraries (Hartford Hospital), **http://www.harthosp.org/library/**

- **Connecticut:** Healthnet: Connecticut Consumer Health Information Center (University of Connecticut Health Center, Lyman Maynard Stowe Library), **http://library.uchc.edu/departm/hnet/**

- **Connecticut:** Waterbury Hospital Health Center Library (Waterbury Hospital), **http://www.waterburyhospital.com/library/consumer.shtml**

- **Delaware:** Consumer Health Library (Christiana Care Health System, Eugene du Pont Preventive Medicine & Rehabilitation Institute), **http://www.christianacare.org/health_guide/health_guide_pmri_health _info.cfm**

- **Delaware:** Lewis B. Flinn Library (Delaware Academy of Medicine), **http://www.delamed.org/chls.html**

- **Georgia:** Family Resource Library (Medical College of Georgia), **http://cmc.mcg.edu/kids_families/fam_resources/fam_res_lib/frl.htm**

- **Georgia:** Health Resource Center (Medical Center of Central Georgia), **http://www.mccg.org/hrc/hrchome.asp**

- **Hawaii:** Hawaii Medical Library: Consumer Health Information Service (Hawaii Medical Library), **http://hml.org/CHIS/**

- **Idaho:** DeArmond Consumer Health Library (Kootenai Medical Center), http://www.nicon.org/DeArmond/index.htm
- **Illinois:** Health Learning Center of Northwestern Memorial Hospital (Northwestern Memorial Hospital, Health Learning Center), http://www.nmh.org/health_info/hlc.html
- **Illinois:** Medical Library (OSF Saint Francis Medical Center), http://www.osfsaintfrancis.org/general/library/
- **Kentucky:** Medical Library - Services for Patients, Families, Students & the Public (Central Baptist Hospital), http://www.centralbap.com/education/community/library.htm
- **Kentucky:** University of Kentucky - Health Information Library (University of Kentucky, Chandler Medical Center, Health Information Library), http://www.mc.uky.edu/PatientEd/
- **Louisiana:** Alton Ochsner Medical Foundation Library (Alton Ochsner Medical Foundation), http://www.ochsner.org/library/
- **Louisiana:** Louisiana State University Health Sciences Center Medical Library-Shreveport, http://lib-sh.lsuhsc.edu/
- **Maine:** Franklin Memorial Hospital Medical Library (Franklin Memorial Hospital), http://www.fchn.org/fmh/lib.htm
- **Maine:** Gerrish-True Health Sciences Library (Central Maine Medical Center), http://www.cmmc.org/library/library.html
- **Maine:** Hadley Parrot Health Science Library (Eastern Maine Healthcare), http://www.emh.org/hll/hpl/guide.htm
- **Maine:** Maine Medical Center Library (Maine Medical Center), http://www.mmc.org/library/
- **Maine:** Parkview Hospital, http://www.parkviewhospital.org/communit.htm#Library
- **Maine:** Southern Maine Medical Center Health Sciences Library (Southern Maine Medical Center), http://www.smmc.org/services/service.php3?choice=10
- **Maine:** Stephens Memorial Hospital Health Information Library (Western Maine Health), http://www.wmhcc.com/hil_frame.html
- **Manitoba, Canada:** Consumer & Patient Health Information Service (University of Manitoba Libraries), http://www.umanitoba.ca/libraries/units/health/reference/chis.html
- **Manitoba, Canada:** J.W. Crane Memorial Library (Deer Lodge Centre), http://www.deerlodge.mb.ca/library/libraryservices.shtml

- **Maryland:** Health Information Center at the Wheaton Regional Library (Montgomery County, Md., Dept. of Public Libraries, Wheaton Regional Library), **http://www.mont.lib.md.us/healthinfo/hic.asp**

- **Massachusetts:** Baystate Medical Center Library (Baystate Health System), **http://www.baystatehealth.com/1024/**

- **Massachusetts:** Boston University Medical Center Alumni Medical Library (Boston University Medical Center), **http://med-libwww.bu.edu/library/lib.html**

- **Massachusetts:** Lowell General Hospital Health Sciences Library (Lowell General Hospital), **http://www.lowellgeneral.org/library/HomePageLinks/WWW.htm**

- **Massachusetts:** Paul E. Woodard Health Sciences Library (New England Baptist Hospital), **http://www.nebh.org/health_lib.asp**

- **Massachusetts:** St. Luke's Hospital Health Sciences Library (St. Luke's Hospital), **http://www.southcoast.org/library/**

- **Massachusetts:** Treadwell Library Consumer Health Reference Center (Massachusetts General Hospital), **http://www.mgh.harvard.edu/library/chrcindex.html**

- **Massachusetts:** UMass HealthNet (University of Massachusetts Medical School), **http://healthnet.umassmed.edu/**

- **Michigan:** Botsford General Hospital Library - Consumer Health (Botsford General Hospital, Library & Internet Services), **http://www.botsfordlibrary.org/consumer.htm**

- **Michigan:** Helen DeRoy Medical Library (Providence Hospital and Medical Centers), **http://www.providence-hospital.org/library/**

- **Michigan:** Marquette General Hospital - Consumer Health Library (Marquette General Hospital, Health Information Center), **http://www.mgh.org/center.html**

- **Michigan:** Patient Education Resouce Center - University of Michigan Cancer Center (University of Michigan Comprehensive Cancer Center), **http://www.cancer.med.umich.edu/learn/leares.htm**

- **Michigan:** Sladen Library & Center for Health Information Resources - Consumer Health Information, **http://www.sladen.hfhs.org/library/consumer/index.html**

- **Montana:** Center for Health Information (St. Patrick Hospital and Health Sciences Center), **http://www.saintpatrick.org/chi/librarydetail.php3?ID=41**

- **National:** Consumer Health Library Directory (Medical Library Association, Consumer and Patient Health Information Section), **http://caphis.mlanet.org/directory/index.html**

- **National:** National Network of Libraries of Medicine (National Library of Medicine) - provides library services for health professionals in the United States who do not have access to a medical library, **http://nnlm.gov/**

- **National:** NN/LM List of Libraries Serving the Public (National Network of Libraries of Medicine), **http://nnlm.gov/members/**

- **Nevada:** Health Science Library, West Charleston Library (Las Vegas Clark County Library District), **http://www.lvccld.org/special_collections/medical/index.htm**

- **New Hampshire:** Dartmouth Biomedical Libraries (Dartmouth College Library), **http://www.dartmouth.edu/~biomed/resources.htmld/conshealth.htmld/**

- **New Jersey:** Consumer Health Library (Rahway Hospital), **http://www.rahwayhospital.com/library.htm**

- **New Jersey:** Dr. Walter Phillips Health Sciences Library (Englewood Hospital and Medical Center), **http://www.englewoodhospital.com/links/index.htm**

- **New Jersey:** Meland Foundation (Englewood Hospital and Medical Center), **http://www.geocities.com/ResearchTriangle/9360/**

- **New York:** Choices in Health Information (New York Public Library) - NLM Consumer Pilot Project participant, **http://www.nypl.org/branch/health/links.html**

- **New York:** Health Information Center (Upstate Medical University, State University of New York), **http://www.upstate.edu/library/hic/**

- **New York:** Health Sciences Library (Long Island Jewish Medical Center), **http://www.lij.edu/library/library.html**

- **New York:** ViaHealth Medical Library (Rochester General Hospital), **http://www.nyam.org/library/**

- **Ohio:** Consumer Health Library (Akron General Medical Center, Medical & Consumer Health Library), **http://www.akrongeneral.org/hwlibrary.htm**

- **Oklahoma:** Saint Francis Health System Patient/Family Resource Center (Saint Francis Health System), **http://www.sfh-tulsa.com/patientfamilycenter/default.asp**

- **Oregon:** Planetree Health Resource Center (Mid-Columbia Medical Center), **http://www.mcmc.net/phrc/**

- **Pennsylvania:** Community Health Information Library (Milton S. Hershey Medical Center), **http://www.hmc.psu.edu/commhealth/**

- **Pennsylvania:** Community Health Resource Library (Geisinger Medical Center), **http://www.geisinger.edu/education/commlib.shtml**

- **Pennsylvania:** HealthInfo Library (Moses Taylor Hospital), **http://www.mth.org/healthwellness.html**

- **Pennsylvania:** Hopwood Library (University of Pittsburgh, Health Sciences Library System), **http://www.hsls.pitt.edu/chi/hhrcinfo.html**

- **Pennsylvania:** Koop Community Health Information Center (College of Physicians of Philadelphia), **http://www.collphyphil.org/kooppg1.shtml**

- **Pennsylvania:** Learning Resources Center - Medical Library (Susquehanna Health System), **http://www.shscares.org/services/lrc/index.asp**

- **Pennsylvania:** Medical Library (UPMC Health System), **http://www.upmc.edu/passavant/library.htm**

- **Quebec, Canada:** Medical Library (Montreal General Hospital), **http://ww2.mcgill.ca/mghlib/**

- **South Dakota:** Rapid City Regional Hospital - Health Information Center (Rapid City Regional Hospital, Health Information Center), **http://www.rcrh.org/education/LibraryResourcesConsumers.htm**

- **Texas:** Houston HealthWays (Houston Academy of Medicine-Texas Medical Center Library), **http://hhw.library.tmc.edu/**

- **Texas:** Matustik Family Resource Center (Cook Children's Health Care System), **http://www.cookchildrens.com/Matustik_Library.html**

- **Washington:** Community Health Library (Kittitas Valley Community Hospital), **http://www.kvch.com/**

- **Washington:** Southwest Washington Medical Center Library (Southwest Washington Medical Center), **http://www.swmedctr.com/Home/**

APPENDIX D. CHILDHOOD SPORTS INJURIES AND THEIR PREVENTION

Overview[28]

The following discussion was prepared by the National Institute of Arthritis and Musculoskeletal and Skin Diseases (NIAMS). It covers the basics of childhood sports injuries and their prevention.

Childhood Sports Injuries and Their Prevention

Childhood sports injuries may be inevitable, but there are some things you can do to help prevent them:

- Enroll your child in organized sports through schools, community clubs, and recreation areas where there may be adults who are certified athletic trainers (ATC). An ATC is also trained in the prevention, recognition and immediate care of athletic injuries.

- Make sure your child uses the proper protective gear for a particular sport. This may lessen the chances of being injured.

- Warm-up exercises, such as stretching and light jogging, can help minimize the chance of muscle strain or other soft tissue injury during sports. Warm-up exercises make the body's tissues warmer and more flexible. Cooling down exercises loosen the body's muscles that have tightened during exercise. Make warm-ups and cool downs part of your child's routine before and after sports participation.

---

[28] Adapted from the National Institute of Arthritis and Musculoskeletal and Skin Diseases (NIAMS): **http://www.niams.nih.gov/hi/topics/childsports/child_sports.htm** .

And don't forget to include sunscreen and a hat (where possible) to reduce the chance of sunburn, which is actually an injury to the skin. Sun protection may also decrease the chances of malignant melanoma--a potentially deadly skin cancer--or other skin cancers that can occur later in life. It is also very important that your child has access to water or a sports drink to stay properly hydrated while playing.

Treat Injuries with "RICE"

If your child receives a soft tissue injury, commonly known as a sprain or a strain, or a bone injury, the best immediate treatment is easy to remember. "RICE" (Rest, Ice, Compression, and Elevation) the injury. Get professional treatment if any injury is severe. A severe injury means having an obvious fracture or dislocation of a joint, prolonged swelling, or prolonged or severe pain.

"RICE"

- **Rest:** Reduce or stop using the injured area for 48 hours. If you have a leg injury, you may need to stay off of it completely.
- **Ice:** Put an ice pack on the injured area for 20 minutes at a time, 4 to 8 times per day. Use a cold pack, ice bag, or a plastic bag filled with crushed ice that has been wrapped in a towel.
- **Compression:** Compression of an injured ankle, knee, or wrist may help reduce the swelling. These include bandages such as elastic wraps, special boots, air casts and splints. Ask your doctor which one is best.
- **Elevation:** Keep the injured area elevated above the level of the heart. Use a pillow to help elevate an injured limb.

Sprains and Strains

A sprain is an injury to a ligament--a stretching or a tearing. One or more ligaments can be injured during a sprain. A ligament is a band of tough, fibrous tissue that connects two or more bones at a joint and prevents excessive movement of the joint. Ankle sprains are the most common injury in the United States and often occur during sports or recreational activities. Approximately 1 million ankle injuries occur each year and 85 percent of these are sprains.

A strain is an injury to either a muscle or a tendon. A muscle is a tissue composed of bundles of specialized cells that, when stimulated by nerve impulses, contract and produce movement. A tendon is a tough, fibrous cord of tissue that connects muscle to bone.

Growth Plate Injuries

In some sports accidents and injuries, the growth plate may be injured. The growth plate is the area of developing tissues at the end of the long bones in growing children and adolescents. When growth is complete, sometime during adolescence, the growth plate is replaced by solid bone. The long bones in the body are the long bones of the fingers, the outer bone of the forearm, the collarbone, the hip, the bone of the upper leg, the lower leg bones, the ankle, and the foot. If any of these areas become injured, seek professional help from a doctor who specializes in bone injuries in children and adolescents (pediatric orthopedist).

Repetitive Motion Injuries

Painful injuries such as stress fractures (where the ligament pulls off small pieces of bone) and tendinitis (inflammation of a tendon) can occur from overuse of muscles and tendons. These injuries don't always show up on x-rays, but they do cause pain and discomfort. The injured area usually responds to rest. Other treatments include RICE, crutches, cast immobilization, or physical therapy.

Heat and Hydration - Playing It Safe Is Cool

Playing rigorous sports in the heat requires close monitoring of both body and weather conditions. Heat injuries are always dangerous and can be fatal. Children perspire less than adults and require a higher core body temperature to trigger sweating. Heat-related illnesses include dehydration (deficit in body fluids), heat exhaustion (nausea, dizziness, weakness, headache, pale and moist skin, heavy perspiration, normal or low body temperature, weak pulse, dilated pupils, disorientation, fainting spells), and heat stroke (headache, dizziness, confusion, and hot dry skin, possibly leading to vascular collapse, coma, and death). These injuries can be prevented.

Playing Safe in the Heat Is Cool

- Recognize the dangers of playing in the heat.
- Respond quickly if heat-related injuries occur.
- Schedule regular fluid breaks during practice and games.
- Drinking water is the best choice; others include fruit juices and sports drinks.
- Kids need to drink 8 ounces of fluid every 20 minutes, plus more after playing.
- Make player substitutions more frequently in the heat.
- Wear light-colored, "breathable" clothing, and wide-brimmed hats
- Use misting water sprays on the body to keep cool.

Exercise Is Beneficial

Even with the risk of injury, your child's involvement in sports is important. Exercise may reduce your child's chances of obesity, which is becoming more common in children. It may also lessen your child's risk of diabetes, a disease that is sometimes associated with a lack of exercise and poor eating habits.

As a parent, it is important for you to match your children to the sport, and not push him or her too hard into an activity that he or she may not like or be capable of doing. Sports also helps children build social skills and provides them with a general sense of well-being. Sports participation is an important part of learning how to build team skills.

Sports Injury and Prevention

You may not be able to protect your child from all sports injuries, but you may be able to reduce the risk of injury by using preventive measures. It is important to know which sports are more likely to cause injury than others. In addition, check the condition of the athletic area where the sports are to be played. Make sure it is properly maintained.
The following "sports scorecard" shows winning ways to help prevent an injury from occurring.

Football

- This popular sport "leads the pack" in the number of injuries, especially in boys, in organized sports.

- Common injuries and locations: Bruises, sprains, strains, pulled muscles, soft tissue tears such as ligaments, broken bones, internal injuries (bruised or damaged organs), back injuries, sunburn. Knees and ankles are the most common injury sites.

- Safest playing with: Helmet; mouth guard; shoulder pads; athletic supporters for males; chest/rib pads; forearm, elbow, and thigh pads; shin guards; proper shoes; sunscreen; water.

- Prevention: Proper use of safety equipment, warm-up exercises, proper coaching and conditioning.

Basketball

- This popular sport has the highest rate of knee injuries requiring surgery among girls.

- Common injuries and locations: Sprains, strains, bruises, fractures, scrapes, dislocation, cuts, dental injuries. Ankles, knees (injury rates are higher in girls, especially for the anterior cruciate ligament, the wide ligament that limits rotation and forward movement of the shin bone), shoulder (rotator cuff strains and tears, where tendons at the end of muscles attach to the upper arm and shoulder bones).

- Safest playing with: Eye protection, elbow and knee pads, mouth guard, athletic supporters for males, proper shoes, water. If playing outdoors, add a hat and sunscreen.

- Prevention: Strength training (particularly knees and shoulders), aerobics (exercises that develop the strength and endurance of heart and lungs), warm-up exercises, proper coaching, and use of safety equipment.

Soccer

- This sport has dramatically increased in popularity in the past two decades in the U.S.

- Common injuries: Bruises, cuts and scrapes, headaches, sunburn.

- Safest playing with: Shin guards, athletic supporters for males, cleats, sunscreen, water.

- Prevention: Aerobic conditioning and warm-ups, and proper training in "heading" the ball. ("Heading" is using the head to strike or make a play with the ball.)

Baseball and Softball

- Sometimes called "America's favorite pastime."
- Common injuries: Soft tissue strains, impact injuries that include fractures due to sliding and being hit by a ball, sunburn.
- Safest playing with: Batting helmet, shin guards, elbow guards, athletic supporters for males, mouth guard, sunscreen, cleats, hat, breakaway bases.
- Prevention: Proper conditioning and warm-ups.

Gymnastics

- The performance of systematic exercises.
- Common injuries: Sprains and strains of soft tissues.
- Safest playing with: Athletic supporters for males, safety harness, joint supports (such as neoprene wraps), water.
- Prevention: Proper conditioning and warm-ups.

Track and Field

- Competing at running, walking, jumping, throwing, or pushing events.
- Common injuries: Strains, sprains, scrapes from falls.
- Safest playing with: Proper shoes, athletic supporters for males, sunscreen, water.
- Prevention: Proper conditioning and coaching.

How Your Child Can Prevent Sports Injuries [29]

- Be in proper physical condition to play the sport.
- Know and abide by the rules of the sport.
- Wear appropriate protective gear (for example, shin guards for soccer, a hard-shell helmet when facing a baseball or softball pitcher, a helmet and body padding for ice hockey).
- Know how to use athletic equipment.
- Always warm up before playing.

---

[29] Adapted from *Play It Safe, a Guide to Safety for Young Athletes,* with permission of the American Academy of Orthopaedic Surgeons.

- Avoid playing when very tired or in pain.

- Get a preseason physical examination.

- Make sure there is adequate water or other liquids to maintain proper hydration.

Additional Resources

For more information on sports injuries and prevention, contact:

National Institute of Arthritis and Musculoskeletal and Skin Diseases
NIAMS/National Institutes of Health
1 AMS Circle
Bethesda, MD 20892-3675
Phone: 301-495-4484; 1-877-22NIAMS (free of charge)
TTY: 301-565-2966
Fax: 301-718-6366
E-mail: NIAMSinfo@mail.nih.gov
www.niams.nih.gov/
NIAMS is a part of the Combined Health Information Database (CHID)
at **http://chid.nih.gov**

Useful NIAMS Links

- Knee Problems: **www.niams.nih.gov/hi/kneeprobs/kneeqa.htm**

- Sprains and Strains:
www.niams.nih.gov/hi/strain_sprain/sprain_strain.htm

- Growth Plate Injuries: **www.naims.nih.gov/hi/growth_plate/growth.htm**

- Shoulder Problems:
www.niams.nih.gov/hi/shoulderprobs/shoulderqa.htm

- NIAMS Information Clearinghouse: **www.niams.nih.gov/hi/**

Other Useful Links

- American Academy of Orthopaedic Surgeons (AAOS): **www.aaos.org**

- American Academy of Pediatrics (AAP): **www.aap.org**

- American College of Rheumatology: **www.rheumatology.org**

- American Medical Society for Sports Medicine (AMSSM): **www.amssm.org**

- American Orthopaedic Society for Sports Medicine (AOSSM): **www.sportsmed.org**
- American Physical Therapy Association (APTA): **www.apta.org**
- Arthritis Foundation (AF): **www.arthritis.org**
- National Athletic Trainers Association (NATA): **www.nata.org**

References

National Athletic Trainers Association. *What happens if your child is injured on the sports field?* Press release. 9/23/99.

O'Connor, Deborah. *Preventing sports injuries in kids.* Patient Care, 6/15/98, pp.60-83.

Powell, John W, Barber-Foss, Kim D. *Injury Patterns in Selected High School Sports: A Review of the 1995-1997 Seasons.* Journal of Athletic Training 1999;34:(3):277-284.

American Academy of Family Physicians. *Heat-Related Illness: What You Can Do to Prevent It.* Brochure. 1994.

Requa, Ralph. *The scope of the problem: the impact of sports-related injuries.* In Proceedings of Sports Injuries in Youth: Surveillance Strategies, Bethesda, MD, 8-9 April 1991. National Institute of Arthritis and Musculoskeletal and Skin Diseases, National Institutes of Health, Bethesda, MD. 11/92, p.19.

Messina, DF; Farney, WC; DeLee, JC. *The incidence of injury in Texas high school basketball.* The American Journal of Sports Medicine. Vol. 27; No.3; 294-299; 1999.

Encyclopedia Britannica Online; **http://members.eb.com**

Vocabulary Builder

Adolescence: The period of life beginning with the appearance of secondary sex characteristics and terminating with the cessation of somatic growth. The years usually referred to as adolescence lie between 13 and 18 years of age. [NIH]

Aerobic: 1. having molecular oxygen present. 2. growing, living, or occurring in the presence of molecular oxygen. 3. requiring oxygen for respiration. [EU]

Ankle: That part of the lower limb directly above the foot. [NIH]

Bandages: Material used for wrapping or binding any part of the body. [NIH]

Collapse: 1. a state of extreme prostration and depression, with failure of circulation. 2. abnormal falling in of the walls of any part of organ. [EU]

Confusion: Disturbed orientation in regard to time, place, or person, sometimes accompanied by disordered consciousness. [EU]

Dehydration: The condition that results from excessive loss of body water. Called also anhydration, deaquation and hypohydration. [EU]

Disorientation: The loss of proper bearings, or a state of mental confusion as to time, place, or identity. [EU]

Dizziness: An imprecise term which may refer to a sense of spatial disorientation, motion of the environment, or lightheadedness. [NIH]

Elastic: Susceptible of resisting and recovering from stretching, compression or distortion applied by a force. [EU]

Fatal: Causing death, deadly; mortal; lethal. [EU]

Hydration: The condition of being combined with water. [EU]

Inflammation: A pathological process characterized by injury or destruction of tissues caused by a variety of cytologic and chemical reactions. It is usually manifested by typical signs of pain, heat, redness, swelling, and loss of function. [NIH]

Malignant: Tending to become progressively worse and to result in death. Having the properties of anaplasia, invasion, and metastasis; said of tumours. [EU]

Melanoma: A tumour arising from the melanocytic system of the skin and other organs. When used alone the term refers to malignant melanoma. [EU]

Nausea: An unpleasant sensation, vaguely referred to the epigastrium and abdomen, and often culminating in vomiting. [EU]

Neoprene: An oil-resistant synthetic rubber made by the polymerization of chloroprene. [NIH]

Pediatrics: A medical specialty concerned with maintaining health and providing medical care to children from birth to adolescence. [NIH]

Perspiration: Sweating; the functional secretion of sweat. [EU]

Pupil: The aperture in the iris through which light passes. [NIH]

Sunburn: An injury to the skin causing erythema, tenderness, and sometimes blistering and resulting from excessive exposure to the sun. The reaction is produced by the ultraviolet radiation in sunlight. [NIH]

ONLINE GLOSSARIES

The Internet provides access to a number of free-to-use medical dictionaries and glossaries. The National Library of Medicine has compiled the following list of online dictionaries:

- ADAM Medical Encyclopedia (A.D.A.M., Inc.), comprehensive medical reference: **http://www.nlm.nih.gov/medlineplus/encyclopedia.html**

- MedicineNet.com Medical Dictionary (MedicineNet, Inc.): **http://www.medterms.com/Script/Main/hp.asp**

- Merriam-Webster Medical Dictionary (Inteli-Health, Inc.): **http://www.intelihealth.com/IH/**

- Multilingual Glossary of Technical and Popular Medical Terms in Eight European Languages (European Commission) - Danish, Dutch, English, French, German, Italian, Portuguese, and Spanish: **http://allserv.rug.ac.be/~rvdstich/eugloss/welcome.html**

- On-line Medical Dictionary (CancerWEB): **http://www.graylab.ac.uk/omd/**

- Technology Glossary (National Library of Medicine) - Health Care Technology: **http://www.nlm.nih.gov/nichsr/ta101/ta10108.htm**

- Terms and Definitions (Office of Rare Diseases): **http://rarediseases.info.nih.gov/ord/glossary_a-e.html**

Beyond these, MEDLINEplus contains a very user-friendly encyclopedia covering every aspect of medicine (licensed from A.D.A.M., Inc.). The ADAM Medical Encyclopedia Web site address is **http://www.nlm.nih.gov/medlineplus/encyclopedia.html**. ADAM is also available on commercial Web sites such as Web MD (**http://my.webmd.com/adam/asset/adam_disease_articles/a_to_z/a**) and drkoop.com (**http://www.drkoop.com/**). Topics of interest can be researched by using keywords before continuing elsewhere, as these basic definitions and concepts will be useful in more advanced areas of research. You may choose to print various pages specifically relating to shoulder separation and keep them on file.

Online Dictionary Directories

The following are additional online directories compiled by the National Library of Medicine, including a number of specialized medical dictionaries and glossaries:

- Medical Dictionaries: Medical & Biological (World Health Organization): **http://www.who.int/hlt/virtuallibrary/English/diction.htm#Medical**

- MEL-Michigan Electronic Library List of Online Health and Medical Dictionaries (Michigan Electronic Library): **http://mel.lib.mi.us/health/health-dictionaries.html**

- Patient Education: Glossaries (DMOZ Open Directory Project): **http://dmoz.org/Health/Education/Patient_Education/Glossaries/**

- Web of Online Dictionaries (Bucknell University): **http://www.yourdictionary.com/diction5.html#medicine**

SHOULDER SEPARATION GLOSSARY

The following is a complete glossary of terms used in this sourcebook. The definitions are derived from official public sources including the National Institutes of Health [NIH] and the European Union [EU]. After this glossary, we list a number of additional hardbound and electronic glossaries and dictionaries that you may wish to consult.

Acromion: The lateral extension of the spine of the scapula and the highest point of the shoulder. [NIH]

Adolescence: The period of life beginning with the appearance of secondary sex characteristics and terminating with the cessation of somatic growth. The years usually referred to as adolescence lie between 13 and 18 years of age. [NIH]

Aerobic: 1. having molecular oxygen present. 2. growing, living, or occurring in the presence of molecular oxygen. 3. requiring oxygen for respiration. [EU]

Ankle: That part of the lower limb directly above the foot. [NIH]

Arthroplasty: Surgical reconstruction of a joint to relieve pain or restore motion. [NIH]

Arthroscopy: Endoscopic examination, therapy and surgery of the joint. [NIH]

Bacteria: Unicellular prokaryotic microorganisms which generally possess rigid cell walls, multiply by cell division, and exhibit three principal forms: round or coccal, rodlike or bacillary, and spiral or spirochetal. [NIH]

Bandages: Material used for wrapping or binding any part of the body. [NIH]

Bursitis: Inflammation of a bursa, occasionally accompanied by a calcific deposit in the underlying supraspinatus tendon; the most common site is the subdeltoid bursa. [EU]

Calcification: The process by which organic tissue becomes hardened by a deposit of calcium salts within its substance. [EU]

Cannula: A tube for insertion into a duct or cavity; during insertion its lumen is usually occupied by a trocar. [EU]

Capsules: Hard or soft soluble containers used for the oral administration of medicine. [NIH]

Carbohydrate: An aldehyde or ketone derivative of a polyhydric alcohol, particularly of the pentahydric and hexahydric alcohols. They are so named because the hydrogen and oxygen are usually in the proportion to form water, $(CH_2O)n$. The most important carbohydrates are the starches, sugars, celluloses, and gums. They are classified into mono-, di-, tri-, poly- and heterosaccharides. [EU]

Cervical: Pertaining to the neck, or to the neck of any organ or structure. [EU]

Cholesterol: The principal sterol of all higher animals, distributed in body tissues, especially the brain and spinal cord, and in animal fats and oils. [NIH]

Chronic: Persisting over a long period of time. [EU]

Collapse: 1. a state of extreme prostration and depression, with failure of circulation. 2. abnormal falling in of the walls of any part of organ. [EU]

Confusion: Disturbed orientation in regard to time, place, or person, sometimes accompanied by disordered consciousness. [EU]

Degenerative: Undergoing degeneration : tending to degenerate; having the character of or involving degeneration; causing or tending to cause degeneration. [EU]

Dehydration: The condition that results from excessive loss of body water. Called also anhydration, deaquation and hypohydration. [EU]

Diarrhea: Passage of excessively liquid or excessively frequent stools. [NIH]

Dislocation: The displacement of any part, more especially of a bone. Called also luxation. [EU]

Disorientation: The loss of proper bearings, or a state of mental confusion as to time, place, or identity. [EU]

Dizziness: An imprecise term which may refer to a sense of spatial disorientation, motion of the environment, or lightheadedness. [NIH]

Dysplasia: Abnormality of development; in pathology, alteration in size, shape, and organization of adult cells. [EU]

Dystocia: Difficult childbirth or labor. [NIH]

Eclampsia: Convulsions and coma occurring in a pregnant or puerperal woman, associated with preeclampsia, i.e., with hypertension, edema, and/or proteinuria. [EU]

Elastic: Susceptible of resisting and recovering from stretching, compression or distortion applied by a force. [EU]

Extremity: A limb; an arm or leg (membrum); sometimes applied specifically to a hand or foot. [EU]

Fatal: Causing death, deadly; mortal; lethal. [EU]

Hemorrhage: Bleeding or escape of blood from a vessel. [NIH]

Hybridization: The genetic process of crossbreeding to produce a hybrid. Hybrid nucleic acids can be formed by nucleic acid hybridization of DNA and RNA molecules. Protein hybridization allows for hybrid proteins to be formed from polypeptide chains. [NIH]

Hydration: The condition of being combined with water. [EU]

Idiopathic: Of the nature of an idiopathy; self-originated; of unknown causation. [EU]

Inflammation: A pathological process characterized by injury or destruction of tissues caused by a variety of cytologic and chemical reactions. It is usually manifested by typical signs of pain, heat, redness, swelling, and loss of function. [NIH]

Intestinal: Pertaining to the intestine. [EU]

Invasive: 1. having the quality of invasiveness. 2. involving puncture or incision of the skin or insertion of an instrument or foreign material into the body; said of diagnostic techniques. [EU]

Iodine: A nonmetallic element of the halogen group that is represented by the atomic symbol I, atomic number 53, and atomic weight of 126.90. It is a nutritionally essential element, especially important in thyroid hormone synthesis. In solution, it has anti-infective properties and is used topically. [NIH]

Kinetic: Pertaining to or producing motion. [EU]

Lesion: Any pathological or traumatic discontinuity of tissue or loss of function of a part. [EU]

Ligament: A band of fibrous tissue that connects bones or cartilages, serving to support and strengthen joints. [EU]

Lumbar: Pertaining to the loins, the part of the back between the thorax and the pelvis. [EU]

Lupus: A form of cutaneous tuberculosis. It is seen predominantly in women and typically involves the nasal, buccal, and conjunctival mucosa. [NIH]

Malignant: Tending to become progressively worse and to result in death. Having the properties of anaplasia, invasion, and metastasis; said of tumours. [EU]

Melanoma: A tumour arising from the melanocytic system of the skin and other organs. When used alone the term refers to malignant melanoma. [EU]

Membrane: A thin layer of tissue which covers a surface, lines a cavity or divides a space or organ. [EU]

Mineralization: The action of mineralizing; the state of being mineralized. [EU]

Mobility: Capability of movement, of being moved, or of flowing freely. [EU]

Molecular: Of, pertaining to, or composed of molecules : a very small mass of matter. [EU]

Morphogenesis: The development of the form of an organ, part of the body, or organism. [NIH]

Nausea: An unpleasant sensation, vaguely referred to the epigastrium and abdomen, and often culminating in vomiting. [EU]

Neonatal: Pertaining to the first four weeks after birth. [EU]

Neoprene: An oil-resistant synthetic rubber made by the polymerization of chloroprene. [NIH]

Neural: 1. pertaining to a nerve or to the nerves. 2. situated in the region of the spinal axis, as the neutral arch. [EU]

Niacin: Water-soluble vitamin of the B complex occurring in various animal and plant tissues. Required by the body for the formation of coenzymes NAD and NADP. Has pellagra-curative, vasodilating, and antilipemic properties. [NIH]

Oral: Pertaining to the mouth, taken through or applied in the mouth, as an oral medication or an oral thermometer. [EU]

Orthopaedic: Pertaining to the correction of deformities of the musculoskeletal system; pertaining to orthopaedics. [EU]

Orthopedics: A surgical specialty which utilizes medical, surgical, and physical methods to treat and correct deformities, diseases, and injuries to the skeletal system, its articulations, and associated structures. [NIH]

Osteoarthritis: Noninflammatory degenerative joint disease occurring chiefly in older persons, characterized by degeneration of the articular cartilage, hypertrophy of bone at the margins, and changes in the synovial membrane. It is accompanied by pain and stiffness, particularly after prolonged activity. [EU]

Overdose: 1. to administer an excessive dose. 2. an excessive dose. [EU]

Palpation: Application of fingers with light pressure to the surface of the body to determine consistence of parts beneath in physical diagnosis; includes palpation for determining the outlines of organs. [NIH]

Pediatrics: A medical specialty concerned with maintaining health and providing medical care to children from birth to adolescence. [NIH]

Perspiration: Sweating; the functional secretion of sweat. [EU]

Phenotype: The outward appearance of the individual. It is the product of interactions between genes and between the genotype and the environment. This includes the killer phenotype, characteristic of yeasts. [NIH]

Posterior: Situated in back of, or in the back part of, or affecting the back or dorsal surface of the body. In lower animals, it refers to the caudal end of the body. [EU]

Potassium: An element that is in the alkali group of metals. It has an atomic symbol K, atomic number 19, and atomic weight 39.10. It is the chief cation in the intracellular fluid of muscle and other cells. Potassium ion is a strong electrolyte and it plays a significant role in the regulation of fluid volume and maintenance of the water-electrolyte balance. [NIH]

Prosthesis: An artificial substitute for a missing body part, such as an arm or leg, eye or tooth, used for functional or cosmetic reasons, or both. [EU]

Proteins: Polymers of amino acids linked by peptide bonds. The specific sequence of amino acids determines the shape and function of the protein. [NIH]

Proximal: Nearest; closer to any point of reference; opposed to distal. [EU]

Pupil: The aperture in the iris through which light passes. [NIH]

Radiography: The making of film records (radiographs) of internal structures of the body by passage of x-rays or gamma rays through the body to act on specially sensitized film. [EU]

Respiratory: Pertaining to respiration. [EU]

Rheumatology: A subspecialty of internal medicine concerned with the study of inflammatory or degenerative processes and metabolic derangement of connective tissue structures which pertain to a variety of musculoskeletal disorders, such as arthritis. [NIH]

Riboflavin: Nutritional factor found in milk, eggs, malted barley, liver, kidney, heart, and leafy vegetables. The richest natural source is yeast. It occurs in the free form only in the retina of the eye, in whey, and in urine; its principal forms in tissues and cells are as FMN and FAD. [NIH]

Selenium: An element with the atomic symbol Se, atomic number 34, and atomic weight 78.96. It is an essential micronutrient for mammals and other animals but is toxic in large amounts. Selenium protects intracellular structures against oxidative damage. It is an essential component of glutathione peroxidase. [NIH]

Spondylitis: Inflammation of the vertebrae. [EU]

Stabilization: The creation of a stable state. [EU]

Sunburn: An injury to the skin causing erythema, tenderness, and sometimes blistering and resulting from excessive exposure to the sun. The reaction is produced by the ultraviolet radiation in sunlight. [NIH]

Surgical: Of, pertaining to, or correctable by surgery. [EU]

Synovial: Of pertaining to, or secreting synovia. [EU]

Systemic: Pertaining to or affecting the body as a whole. [EU]

Tendinitis: Inflammation of tendons and of tendon-muscle attachments. [EU]

Thermoregulation: Heat regulation. [EU]

Thyroxine: An amino acid of the thyroid gland which exerts a stimulating effect on thyroid metabolism. [NIH]

Tolerance: 1. the ability to endure unusually large doses of a drug or toxin. 2. acquired drug tolerance; a decreasing response to repeated constant doses of a drug or the need for increasing doses to maintain a constant response. [EU]

Tomography: The recording of internal body images at a predetermined plane by means of the tomograph; called also body section roentgenography. [EU]

Toxic: Pertaining to, due to, or of the nature of a poison or toxin; manifesting the symptoms of severe infection. [EU]

General Dictionaries and Glossaries

While the above glossary is essentially complete, the dictionaries listed here cover virtually all aspects of medicine, from basic words and phrases to more advanced terms (sorted alphabetically by title; hyperlinks provide rankings, information and reviews at Amazon.com):

- **Dictionary of Medical Acronymns & Abbreviations** by Stanley Jablonski (Editor), Paperback, 4th edition (2001), Lippincott Williams & Wilkins Publishers, ISBN: 1560534605, **http://www.amazon.com/exec/obidos/ASIN/1560534605/icongroupinterna**

- **Dictionary of Medical Terms : For the Nonmedical Person (Dictionary of Medical Terms for the Nonmedical Person, Ed 4)** by Mikel A. Rothenberg, M.D, et al, Paperback - 544 pages, 4th edition (2000), Barrons Educational Series, ISBN: 0764112015, **http://www.amazon.com/exec/obidos/ASIN/0764112015/icongroupinterna**

- **A Dictionary of the History of Medicine** by A. Sebastian, CD-Rom edition (2001), CRC Press-Parthenon Publishers, ISBN: 185070368X, **http://www.amazon.com/exec/obidos/ASIN/185070368X/icongroupinterna**

- **Dorland's Illustrated Medical Dictionary (Standard Version)** by Dorland, et al, Hardcover - 2088 pages, 29th edition (2000), W B Saunders Co, ISBN: 0721662544, **http://www.amazon.com/exec/obidos/ASIN/0721662544/icongroupinterna**

- **Dorland's Electronic Medical Dictionary** by Dorland, et al, Software, 29th Book & CD-Rom edition (2000), Harcourt Health Sciences, ISBN: 0721694934, **http://www.amazon.com/exec/obidos/ASIN/0721694934/icongroupinterna**

- **Dorland's Pocket Medical Dictionary (Dorland's Pocket Medical Dictionary, 26th Ed)** Hardcover - 912 pages, 26th edition (2001), W B Saunders Co, ISBN: 0721682812, http://www.amazon.com/exec/obidos/ASIN/0721682812/icongroupinterna /103-4193558-7304618

- **Melloni's Illustrated Medical Dictionary (Melloni's Illustrated Medical Dictionary, 4th Ed)** by Melloni, Hardcover, 4th edition (2001), CRC Press-Parthenon Publishers, ISBN: 85070094X, http://www.amazon.com/exec/obidos/ASIN/85070094X/icongroupinterna

- **Stedman's Electronic Medical Dictionary Version 5.0 (CD-ROM for Windows and Macintosh, Individual)** by Stedmans, CD-ROM edition (2000), Lippincott Williams & Wilkins Publishers, ISBN: 0781726328, http://www.amazon.com/exec/obidos/ASIN/0781726328/icongroupinterna

- **Stedman's Medical Dictionary** by Thomas Lathrop Stedman, Hardcover - 2098 pages, 27th edition (2000), Lippincott, Williams & Wilkins, ISBN: 068340007X, http://www.amazon.com/exec/obidos/ASIN/068340007X/icongroupinterna

- **Tabers Cyclopedic Medical Dictionary (Thumb Index)** by Donald Venes (Editor), et al, Hardcover - 2439 pages, 19th edition (2001), F A Davis Co, ISBN: 0803606540, http://www.amazon.com/exec/obidos/ASIN/0803606540/icongroupinterna

INDEX

A
Acromion 11, 12
Adolescence 79, 84, 85, 89, 92
Ankle................................ 78, 79
Arthroplasty 38, 46
Arthroscopy 14, 45
B
Bacteria 60
Bandages 78
Bursitis 17, 32
C
Calcification 32
Cannula...44
Capsules 63
Carbohydrate...................................62
Cervical 12
Cholesterol 60, 62
Chronic...17
Collapse 79
Confusion 79, 85, 90
D
Degenerative 12, 19, 33, 61, 92, 93
Dehydration 79
Diarrhea 60
Dislocation 10, 17, 32, 46, 78, 81
Disorientation.........................79, 85, 90
Dizziness..79
Dystocia 17, 46
E
Eclampsia..17
Elastic 78
Extremity 36
F
Fatal...79
H
Hemorrhage.......................................17
Hydration 83
I
Inflammation 79
Intestinal...60
Invasive..13
L
Ligament 78, 79, 81

Lupus 65
M
Malignant 78, 85, 91
Melanoma 78, 85, 91
Membrane..............................11, 33, 92
Mobility...12
Molecular 84, 89
N
Nausea 79
Neoprene 82
Neural 61
Niacin..61
O
Oral...............................33, 67, 89, 92
Orthopaedic............................... 10, 37
Osteoarthritis 32
Overdose 61
P
Palpation................................32, 34, 92
Perspiration 79
Phenotype 34, 92
Posterior..46
Potassium 62
Prosthesis 45
Proteins 33, 60, 62, 90
Proximal..45
R
Rheumatology 14, 83
Riboflavin 60
S
Selenium 62, 65
Sunburn 78, 81, 82
Surgical 13, 38, 44, 45, 47, 92
Synovial 11, 33, 92
Systemic 65
T
Tears 44, 45, 81
Tendinitis................................... 32, 79
Thermoregulation...............................60
Thyroxine 62
Tolerance 41, 94
Tomography 32
Toxic......................................61, 68, 93

Printed in the United States
899100001B

9 780597 831768